Women's Health

A practical guide to all the stages
and ages of the female life cycle

Gillian McKeith

'With love to my Mum and daughters.'

MICHAEL JOSEPH

Published by the Penguin Group
Penguin Books Ltd, 80 Strand, London WC2R 0RL, England
Penguin Group (USA) Inc., 375 Hudson Street, New York, New York 10014, USA
Penguin Group (Canada), 90 Eglinton Avenue East, Suite 700, Toronto, Ontario, Canada M4P 2Y3
(a division of Pearson Penguin Canada Inc.)
Penguin Ireland, 25 St Stephen's Green, Dublin 2, Ireland (a division of Penguin Books Ltd)
Penguin Group (Australia), 250 Camberwell Road,
Camberwell, Victoria 3124, Australia (a division of Pearson Australia Group Pty Ltd)
Penguin Books India Pvt Ltd, 11 Community Centre,
Panchsheel Park, New Delhi – 110 017, India
Penguin Group (NZ), 67 Apollo Drive, Rosedale, North Shore 0632, New Zealand
(a division of Pearson New Zealand Ltd)
Penguin Books (South Africa) (Pty) Ltd, 24 Sturdee Avenue,
Rosebank, Johannesburg 2196, South Africa

Penguin Books Ltd, Registered Offices: 80 Strand, London WC2R 0RL, England

www.penguin.com

Published in 2010

1

Copyright © Gillian McKeith, 2010

The moral right of the author has been asserted

Printed in China

A CIP catalogue record for this book is available from the British Library

ISBN: 978-0-718-15435-6

Contents

A celebration of womanhood

Welcome to our celebration of womanhood. My mission is to empower you to be a fit, happy, sexy, healthy female, whatever your age.

I contend that women are the most amazing creatures! We handle anything and everything, we do so much, we hold the family together, which means we hold the world together. And, quite frankly, if it wasn't for us females there would be no 'next generation'. We multi-task, we bring life, new babies, we work, keep the house in order, we knit, some of us even bake cookies, we are soldiers and leaders too, and some of us run companies and countries as well. We have the ability to do it all. So don't let anyone diss women!

I am not down on men; I love men, fancy too many of them and sometimes even admire them. But women often get a bum rap in the PR department. We've all heard about 'women's problems', 'a woman's lot', 'wait till you get your period', 'hormonal hell...' and on it goes. How often do we hear these negative phrases flying around when it comes to our gender's health? The other day, my own nine-year-old daughter said unexpectedly to my husband, 'Daddy, you're so lucky that you're not a lady, because you don't get a period or have to go through childbirth.' Wow, where did that come from?! I am here to debunk those age-old stereotypes, because I don't buy into them. I have been consulting with private clients for almost twenty years, both males and females, and I am here to assure you that women have a wonderful physiological system to enjoy, cherish and, yes, celebrate. Let's not think of ourselves as cursed – we certainly are not. The fact is that we women are all truly special. And this book honours that 'specialness'.

But if you're someone who has experienced painful or heavy periods, or chronic PMS, or hot flushes, say, you're probably reading this and telling me to get real! Before you throw the book across the room, let me tell you that my optimism is founded on experience. My many years of working with women and their wellbeing have proved to me that you can relieve, eliminate, manage or prevent many or most ills and common complaints with good nutrition, change of lifestyle and a willing mindset.

More than 75 per cent of my clients tend to be female. Of my male clients, most of them came to see me originally because their wives, mothers or sisters sent them; so the point here is that we women actually do care about our health – how we feel and look – as well as the health of our men. We know it's important to be proactive and protect ourselves from disease. And we know that what we eat and how we live our lives has a huge influence on how we look and feel on a day-to-day basis. The problem is that we don't always put this knowledge into practice, because either we think we're too tired or just too busy. We often forget about ourselves. Instead we are focused on the wellbeing and the nurturing of our kids, our partners, spouses, parents, siblings and even friends. It's easy to lose yourself. When I was a youngster, I used to hear some older people say, 'I want to find myself.' And I would just laugh, wondering, 'Where did they get lost?' Once you are a mum, you definitely know what it means to lose yourself and want to find 'you' again. It's not just mothers who are at risk of losing themselves, it's everyone who loses focus on who they really are. This book will allow you as a woman to find the real you, to focus on you and make yourself a priority as you should be.

'It is impossible to nurture another person if you don't nurture yourself first and foremost.'

I imagine that you'll have certain expectations about this book. Yes, it's a health book that's based on good nutrition so, sure enough, we will be talking a lot about the right foods to eat and supplements to take – and why – to optimize your health as a woman.

But I've been working in the field of nutrition for many years now and my work has evolved to include so, so much more – which I want to pass on to you, too. The key to my life's work is that I focus on physical and metaphysical energies in life. The physical is that which you perceive, that you can easily see, taste and smell. The metaphysical is that which you cannot. And I believe that merging the two together – giving them equal importance in life – is what will really take your health to new heights. Let me explain further...

When I talk about physical energy, I'm talking about food. What you eat and drink provides you with living, physical energy on a day-to-day basis. It's essential for life. It provides fuel for energy, repairs your cells, fights infection, controls hormones, staves off stress... And it's what you eat, and how, that can influence how well your body performs all these functions, and how fantastic you may feel. Energies vibrate at different rates and food of the highest nutritional quality vibrates with the highest vibrational energy. It'll come as no surprise, then, that this is the type of food I encourage you to eat! A good diet and lifestyle, with high-energy foods, along with herbs, occasional supplements and natural therapies, have the power to heal, nurture and rejuvenate you. This makes up the physical side of my work.

So what do I mean by the metaphysical? Well, it's quite simple really – and anyone who gives any thought to being mentally and emotionally healthy is already, without perhaps knowing, working on their metaphysical energy.

Your thoughts, feelings, emotions and spirit make up your metaphysical energy which, like the physical energy provided by food, also vibrates. And the two interact. When all of your energies, physical and metaphysical, are properly synchronized, you then feel well, look great, are in good spirits and you then stay well, too. OK, illness may strike from time to time, but you'll be far better equipped to fight it. Another way of putting it is that optimum health is not just about what you put inside yourself; it's about your attitude, actions, responses – how you live, breathe and feel your life.

In this book, I will help you to discover how to synchronize your energy, on both these physical and metaphysical levels. There will be a specific energy exercise for each life stage, which will help you to develop your skills for energy synchronization. These involve methods such as breathing techniques, visualization, self-hypnosis, meditation and more. They'll help you to work with your own healing energies and release deep emotions and mental blocks that may hinder your health. Give them a go – even if you're not sure at first. I promise you'll soon find they become valuable life skills – all my clients tell me so!

This book is firmly grounded in the specific concerns of women. And you will get results for a lifetime. I deal with the main issues for ladies that I come across in my own practice as I know how significant they are for you. I give you my practical advice on being the best you can be and harnessing good health at any and all ages in order to realize your potential.

This is a reference handbook for all women throughout their lives.

Wishing you love and light,

Gillian

How to use this book

Gillian McKeith's *Women's Health* provides you with the necessary information to embark on a holistic approach to protecting against, helping to alleviate or sorting out a raft of common ailments so that you feel your healthiest, sexiest and happiest throughout life. The book is divided into four main sections, each corresponding with a female life stage:

1 Puberty

2 Reproductive years

3 Perimenopause

4 Post-menopause and beyond

You may choose to read this book from cover to cover, or you may prefer to consult only the section which corresponds with your current life stage. But I urge you to use it as a reference guide always. Share it with your teenage daughter or niece, show it to your mum, your sister or any other female you care about. It's for all of you.

Each section talks through my nutritional and lifestyle advice for how to be the best that you can be, highlighting specific areas of your health to focus on. I then move on to the common ailments most likely to occur in that life stage. I explain what they are and what you can do about them. In effect, I write you my nutritional prescription for each common complaint.

I have divided up these common ailments to sit in the life stage where they most commonly occur. For example, Premenstrual Syndrome can be found in the Puberty section. That's not to say, of course, that you won't experience PMS in your reproductive or perimenopausal years as well, and the advice I give is relevant whatever your age.

Gillian McKeith's 10 principles to empower every woman

1 **DIRECT INFLUENCE:** You have direct influence on your health and wellbeing when you take control of your life. As a woman you must take responsibility for your health. It should not matter how old you are: whether young, middle-aged or elderly, it is never too late to take control. You can always make a positive shift, even if it's just incremental bits at a time. I want you to become a proactive planner for your life. Make conscious decisions about what you put into your body, when and how you move your body and everything else that you do in your life. Once you empower yourself, this principle has implications in all realms of your person: the physical, the emotional, the financial and the spiritual aspects. You are the one deciding how to move forward with your life.

Some of my clients have complained that just the thought of taking control is too overwhelming and exhausting. It's yet another thing they have to do. They tell me this will send them 'over the edge'. It does not work that way. When you actually do take control, you will find that you feel less overwhelmed, less tired, calmer and more grounded. But you must take that first leap.

2 **INTERNAL PEACE:** Internal peace brings harmony to your physical, psychological, emotional and spiritual self. This is easy to achieve. Internal peace comes when you calm the mind and let go of all the chatter in your head. At first, this might sound like a monumental task but I will show you how to achieve internal peace.

First of all, sit in a chair with your bare feet firmly on the floor. Feel your feet touching the ground. Imagine you have roots going down your legs through your feet into the floor. Sit comfortably in silence in a quiet room. Notice your body and skin. Then pay attention to your breathing. Take note how the breath enters your body and fills up your legs, feet, tummy, chest, back, head and arms. Imagine that you are able to literally watch how your breath leaves the body. Keep listening and watching your breath as it slowly goes in and out of your body.

Do this for five minutes every day. The reality is that you are not actually doing anything; rather, you are simply watching and listening to your own breathing. If you do this simple exercise every day, you will start to experience an inner peace in all realms of yourself.

3   **SELF LOVE:** The energetic vibration of self love, gratitude, joy and love for ALL delivers harmony to the human condition. I have spent many years consulting in private practice with female clients who hated themselves. So many women nowadays don't like the way they look, their body shape or are worried about their weight. I can definitely tell you that the biggest problem I deal with is self hate.

At the moment, I actually have five women who, when they first started coming to me, told me that they hated themselves. One lady would look at herself in the mirror each day and would repeatedly say: 'I hate you. I am ugly.' Another woman could not even bear to look at herself in the mirror because she told me she was 'too gross'.

I am now going to disclose one of the greatest secrets to you loud and clear. Self love and the energy of love itself is the highest healing frequency that exists. By tapping into your inner love that rests within yourself, you then bring inner harmony to your Being.

We are now going to tell our brain, body and soul that we actually love ourselves:

Each day look in the mirror, look at all of you. Listen and take note of your breathing as you calm your mind. Continue to look at yourself in the mirror and notice your breathing. While looking in the mirror, say to yourself: 'I love me. I love all of me. I love all of life. I am a beautiful person.' Now give yourself a peck on the lips in the mirror.

4 **HARMONY:** Fostering inner harmony is essential healing energy for total wellness on all levels.

When your body is in balance with itself and its surroundings, then you can adapt to almost anything; it is at ease. Fostering inner harmony requires a full-spectrum approach. In this way, you balance yourself on all levels: physical, mental, emotional and spiritual.

Here's how it works: First, nourish your physical body with pure food. Second, nourish your mind with pure thoughts. This means that you constantly feed your mind with thoughts that are happy, positive, favourable and healthy. Third, nourish your emotions by allowing yourself to recognize how you feel; acknowledge head-on the emotions you are experiencing. Allow the emotions to flow through you and ultimately away. Let go. Fourth, nourish your spirit through quiet breathing and meditation exercises that allow you to calm the mind so that you can feel, enter and experience your soul in its truest form.

5 **BALANCE:** Inner personal balance can further render harmony to others: family, neighbours, community and the world.

When you are out of balance in any aspect of your life, it can affect those around you adversely and create a type of imbalance and chaos in all directions. Imagine if your boss walked into a quiet stable office and started shouting and raging about something or other. What would happen? Workers would feel very unnerved, possibly disoriented, some would get angry and probably be unable to work. But if the same boss were to walk into that same office in a state of absolute peace, calm and harmony, all of the office workers will not only feel and absorb those harmonic energies, but undoubtedly the work from that office would be smoother, better and more expansive. In effect, if you can create a state of inner balance, then you vibrate to others what state of being you are in. A state of balance is achieved by:

- physical nourishment

- calming the mind with exercises like meditation and listening to breath

- physical movements like chi gung, yoga, stretching and walking

6 **THANKS:** Give thanks each day for the Trinity of Life: Self, Earth, Universe.
Gratitude and appreciation are the most important energies for health and wellness.

When waking in the morning and retiring at night, offer appreciation. Stand in a quiet space. Extend your arms from side to side with open palms and say, 'Thank you to the Universe.' Now take both palms, hold them against your chest around your heart region and say, 'Thank you for me.' Place your hands in prayer position with both palms touching and say, 'Thank you for the earth and all life.' Lower your head and bow in gratitude. That's all you need to say and do.

7 **ENERGIES:** All elements within and outside our consciousness are energies that affect our health and wellbeing.
Your thoughts, words and actions all have an influence on your body's health and wellbeing; your thoughts, words and

actions also impact on your interactions and relationships with others. Think of a boomerang: what you put out there comes back to you with greater force. When you gossip nastily about another or think negative thoughts about someone or commit deliberately lousy actions, you are creating toxins within your own body. In effect, you are polluting your mind, body and spirit. When someone disparages or defames another person, they are also rubbishing themselves. Make your thoughts, words and actions pure and positive.

8 **FOOD AND WATER:** Food and water are the most basic and essential physical energies that affect our bodies. All foods carry a vibrational charge. Our vitality comes from the foods we eat. The vitality of a food can also be described in terms of its vibration. The higher the vibration, the higher the vitality and the more life-giving the foods are. I want you to eat foods that have good energy. Unadulterated food from nature in its original form is the fuel that powers your life. From a human health standpoint, good food motivates good energy and thus delivers good health to your body. Be open to eating not only new good foods but also a wide variety of foods.

If you feed your body with processed, empty calories, chemically tainted and additive-filled foods, high in white sugar, lacking in fibre with low-vibrational frequency, then you will feel the negative effects. If you eat high-vibrational food, you will feel better. Know this: There is a direct connection between what you put into your body and how you feel.

Your organs, brain and hormones could not function without water. Water is vital for oxygenating the cells, removing wastes and regulating temperature. Good hydration is essential for preventing so many conditions, including urinary tract disorders, constipation, high blood pressure, cardiovascular disease, impaired cognitive function, dental disease, gallstones and glaucoma. Dehydration can impair physical and cognitive performance, including alertness, memory and ability to concentrate.

9   **BREATHING:** Breathing can free up blockages and directly impact on our health and vitality.
Getting the body's internal energy flowing is essential to start the healing process. Once the energy is flowing freely the body's own healing mechanisms can come into play. Oxygen is a vital part of this process; breathing exercises that increase tissue oxygenation and exhalation of toxins are cleansing and revitalizing. For this reason, in each section of this book I include an energy-balancing practice which starts and ends with a focus on your breathing.

10   **INNER POWER:** We have the power to support our own healing and rejuvenate ourselves and each other with our own harmonized physical and metaphysical vibrational energy. If we are in balance, then we bring peace to ourselves and those around us. Believe in yourself and your inner power.

Your health status: it's quiz time

I wish I had a mung bean for every client who's ever said, 'Oh, I'm pretty healthy really...', then gone on to give me a list of ailments as long as their arm. I could make mung-bean stew for the whole of Scotland for generations to come.

It's the same if I ask people to fill in a food and exercise diary for a week or two. You see, they believe they eat well, they really do. But the truth, on paper, tells a different story. 'I never realized I drank so much coffee/had takeaways that often/only exercised twice a month...' comes the familiar cry.

I agree it can be hard to assess your own health status. Unless you've ever felt your absolute best – full of life and positive energy and symptom-free – how do you know how far you've got to go to get there?

That's why I've devised these simple quizzes for the four life stages I cover in this book. Take the quiz that's relevant to you, and you'll get a good general idea of how well you're doing and how big a transformation you need to make. If you have the time, I can highly recommend keeping that food, mood and exercise diary for at least a week before you do the quiz. That way you'll get a more truthful picture of your diet and lifestyle habits.

Have fun!

QUIZ 1: Puberty

Score each of the following questions from 0–5:
0 = never
1–2 = occasionally
3–4 = often
5 = regularly, always or chronically

1. Do you suffer from PMS symptoms such as irritability, cravings, breast tenderness or mood swings, arguing with your mum and family?

2. Are your periods heavy or irregular?

3. Do you regularly suffer from thrush or cystitis?

4. Do you regularly suffer from spots or skin outbreaks?

5. Do you lack energy or lose concentration easily?

6. Is your diet high in soft drinks, chocolates, biscuits, cakes and sweets?

7. Do you drink alcohol, smoke or use other drugs?

8. Do you crave sugar and refined carbohydrates?

9. Do you tend to eat irregularly?

10. Do you engage in physical activity less than three times a week?

How did you score?

0 – Excellent, you're a girl after my own heart! It sounds as if you're doing many of the right things in terms of looking after your body and balancing your female hormones. This will stand you in good stead during your reproductive years. Keep up the good work, but if there are any conditions you know your female relatives suffer from, then do read up on them.

1–5 – You may have slight hormonal imbalance somewhere along the line. And it's always best to nip problems in the bud before they take hold. Many imbalances and their symptoms can be corrected by eating a good diet, balancing blood sugar and taking regular exercise. Pay attention to your intake of essential fats, magnesium, zinc and B6 as these are all vital for female hormones.

6–10 – Most female hormonal imbalances can be corrected fairly easily. Someone as young as you can almost certainly take some fairly simple steps to correct your imbalances. It is likely that your blood-sugar levels are unstable and this can have a negative effect on your female hormones. Avoiding sugary foods and refined carbohydrates is essential. Making these sorts of changes to your diet and taking some exercise can make a huge difference to how you feel.

11–20 – You're probably aware things aren't quite right with your health at this stage. Don't panic – you don't need to feel like this, and there are lots of things I can teach you to help restore hormonal balance. Read the sections that are relevant to you. Taking in the right nutrients, avoiding hormone disrupters and doing daily exercise and relaxation could help to ease your symptoms.

Over 20 – OK, let's talk turkey here. Things need to change and pronto. There are a number of dietary and lifestyle changes you could make that will have you feeling a whole lot better. I can't stress enough that it's important to nourish and support your system as much as possible now to avoid further complications later in life. Cut out sugary foods and drinks. Replace white, refined foods with whole grains. Read the sections that are relevant to you and begin to follow the recommendations as soon as you can. If I could invite you to stay at my house for a month-long health boot camp, I would. You need it! Luckily this book will help you to help yourself.

QUIZ 2: Your reproductive years

Score each of the following questions from 0–5:
0 = never
1–2 = occasionally
3–4 = often
5 = regularly, always or chronically

1. Do you suffer from PMS symptoms such as irritability, cravings, breast tenderness or mood swings?

2. Are your periods irregular or heavy?

3. Does your menstrual cycle last for fewer than 22 days?

4. Have you ever tried to become pregnant without success?

5. Do you suffer from a diminished libido?

6. Have you ever had a miscarriage?

7. Have you had a sexually transmitted infection (STI) in the past two years?

8. Do you suffer from thrush or cystitis?

9. Have you ever been diagnosed with any condition associated with the sex hormones or reproductive system, such as PCOS, endometriosis, fibrocystic breast disease, ovarian cysts, fibroids or cancer of the cervix, breast or ovaries?

10. Do you carry weight around your breasts, hips or bum that you find hard to shift?

How did you score?

0 – I'm impressed! It sounds as if your reproductive system is in a pretty good state of health and your female hormones are well balanced. Keep up the good work but do read up on any conditions that run in your family. And remember, good health can always be enhanced, so keep trying new foods and ways to nourish yourself.

1–5 – Pretty good but it sounds as if there may be a slight imbalance somewhere along the line. It is always best to nip problems in the bud. Read up on any sections that are relevant to your symptoms. Pay attention to your intake of essential fats, magnesium, zinc and B6 as these are all vital for a healthy reproductive system.

6–10 – Making some changes to your nutritional status through diet and supplements, along with a few lifestyle changes, could help to reduce your symptoms, if not eliminate them altogether. You could feel so much better than you do! Read the relevant sections and start following the recommendations immediately.

11–20 – You probably realize that your female hormones may be out of balance. Your lifestyle needs a good overhaul and you know it. Read the sections that are relevant to you to help to restore balance. Taking in the right nutrients, avoiding hormone disrupters and making time for daily exercise and relaxation could help to improve your symptoms. In fact, I know it will!

Over 20 – Thank goodness you're reading my book, because you need help! You may well have been suffering with your symptoms for quite some time. However, they're not your destiny, there is a way forward. So many conditions of the female reproductive system can be improved through diet and lifestyle techniques, believe me. Read the sections that are relevant to you and begin to follow the recommendations as soon as you can.

QUIZ 3: The perimenopause

Score each of the following questions from 0–5:
0 = never
1–2 = occasionally
3–4 = often
5 = regularly, always or chronically

1. Do you have less energy than you used to or do you tire easily?

2. Do you suffer from vaginal dryness or dry skin?

3. Is your sex drive lower than you'd like?

4. Are you overweight or do you tend to put on weight easily and find it hard to shift?

5. Are you gaining more weight around your middle than usual?

6. Do you feel light-headed or irritable if you don't eat regularly?

7. Does you hair seem to be getting thinner?

8. Do you suffer from hot flushes or night sweats?

9. Are you experiencing mood swings, emotional volatility, anxiety or depression?

10. Have your periods become heavy, irregular or painful or do they seem to have stopped?

How did you score?

0 – Congratulations. It sounds as if you are doing many of the right things in terms of looking after your body – you may be one of those women who simply sails through the menopause with nothing bad to report. Keep up the good work, but if there are any conditions from which your female relatives have suffered, then read the relevant sections on them. Forewarned is forearmed!

1–5 – You're pretty healthy and balanced, but it's never too late to improve your diet and lifestyle. Eating a good diet, balancing blood sugar and taking regular exercise may help to even out the hormonal fluctuations that may be causing minor symptoms. Pay attention to your intake of essential fats, magnesium and zinc as these are all vital for health and may not feature enough in your diet.

6–10 – It is likely that there are a few imbalances in your system – best to deal with them sooner rather than later. The transitional stage through to menopause does not need to be a difficult time health-wise. Avoiding sugary foods, refined carbohydrates, caffeine and alcohol can be really helpful as these foods can all have a negative effect on the hormonal system. Making these sorts of changes to your diet and taking some exercise can make a huge difference to how you feel both now and in the future.

11–20 – The perimenopause may be hitting you harder than it needs to. There are lots of steps you can take to help to counter the effects of hormonal changes that naturally take place at this time of life. Plant oestrogens, essential fats, magnesium and B vitamins can all be extremely useful. There are also many herbs that have been used for centuries to support women through the menopause and beyond, and they'll help you, too!

Over 20 – Right, you've suffered enough – this stops here! There are significant dietary and lifestyle changes you could make that will help you start to enjoy this time of your life. It's important to nourish and support your system as much as possible. Apart from helping with the hormonal fluctuations, dietary and lifestyle changes made now could help you to avoid health problems later in life. This would be a good time to cut out sugary foods and drinks and to replace white, refined foods with whole grains. Read the sections that are relevant to you and begin to follow my recommendations without delay.

QUIZ 4: Post-menopause and beyond

Score each of the following questions from 0–5:
0 = never
1–2 = occasionally
3–4 = often
5 = regularly, always or chronically

1. Do you tire at the slightest exertion or experience shortness of breath regularly?

2. Are you overweight or do you tend to put on weight easily and find it hard to shift?

3. Do you have excess weight around your middle or have you been diagnosed with diabetes or metabolic syndrome?

4. Have you been diagnosed with high blood pressure, high cholesterol or cardiovascular problems?

5. Are you becoming increasingly forgetful?

6. Are you experiencing aches, pains or inflammation in any parts of your body?

7. Do you suffer from depression, anxiety or insomnia?

8. Have you fractured any bones in the past few years or been diagnosed with brittle bones or osteoporosis?

9. Do you avoid exercise or spend most of your time sitting down?

10. Are you compromised in terms of what you can eat due to dental health, digestive problems or trouble preparing foods?

How did you score?

0 – You are indeed a wise woman! Years of experience have taught you how best to look after your body. And you'll feel the benefits over the coming decades if you keep up the good work. Do take the time to find out if there are any health conditions from which your relatives have suffered, then read the relevant sections. And don't neglect your self-checks, screening and diagnostic tests.

1–5 – You're healthy enough to be an inspiration to most of your contemporaries, I'm sure. So carry on inspiring them by improving your diet and lifestyle even more. Any health niggles you do have can doubtless be corrected by eating a good diet, balancing blood sugar and taking regular exercise. Pay attention to your intake of essential fats, magnesium, zinc and B vitamins as these nutrients may well help to prevent many health problems.

6–10 – It is likely that there are a few imbalances in your system that are best dealt with sooner rather than later. Avoiding sugary foods and refined carbohydrates is essential. Spend time trying healthy recipes and new foods that you can prepare easily. Taking some exercise and getting some fresh air every day can make a huge difference to how you feel both now and in the future.

11–20 – Sounds as if you're feeling a little out of sorts. Yet there are still lots of things you could do to help to restore balance to your system even if you have fairly long-term symptoms or existing illnesses. Read the sections that are relevant to you. Taking in the right nutrients and daily exercise and relaxation could help to improve your wellbeing and prevent any deterioration.

Over 20 – It's never too late to change your habits. There are a number of dietary and lifestyle changes you can make today that will change the way you feel for the better. It is important to nourish and support your system as much as possible now to avoid further complications. This would be a good time to cut out sugary foods and drinks and to replace white, refined foods with whole grains. Read the sections that are relevant to you and begin to follow the recommendations as soon as you can. Seek help with shopping and preparing foods if you are struggling with these aspects of healthy eating.

The female hormones

My experience with clients is that most women know the *names* of the female hormones but, well, they're not entirely sure what they *do*. So, as we're going to be talking a lot about female hormones in this book, here's a quick guide.

Your ovaries produce the steroid hormones, oestrogen and progesterone. It is the monthly fluctuations of these two hormones that cause the female menstrual cycle of ovulation and menstruation. It is important that oestrogen and progesterone are in balance with each other as if one or other is dominant symptoms of PMS, irregular or heavy periods, or other problems with the reproductive system can result.

The hormone oestrogen

WHAT IT IS While we tend to think of oestrogen as being one substance, it is actually the name for a family of hormones, of which there are three main types. These are oestradiol, oestriol and oestrone. Oestradiol is the main type in non-pregnant females. Oestriol is the main type during pregnancy. And oestrone is higher during the menopause.

WHAT IT DOES Oestrogen is responsible for female sexual characteristics such as breast development and widening hips. It increases libido, particularly around ovulation. It also thins the cervical mucus which makes it easier for sperm to travel further, and stimulates growth of the endometrium (your womb lining) in preparation for a fertilized egg. Oestrogen also multitasks by: increasing skin elasticity, stimulating the production of High Density Lipoproteins (HDL or 'good' cholesterol) and helping to keep bones healthy. When out of balance it may also increase salt and fluid retention.

The hormone progesterone

WHAT IT IS The key hormone of pregnancy

WHAT IT DOES Progesterone prepares the body for pregnancy and helps to maintain the pregnancy. It then plays a part in stimulating the breasts to prepare for milk production. It thickens the cervical mucus, making it more difficult for sperm to get through. Like oestrogen, it stimulates the creation of new bone cells, protecting against osteoporosis. And it balances salt and fluid levels by increasing their loss from the body.

The hormone gonadotrophin

WHAT IT IS Gonadotrophins are hormones that stimulate the gonads – the ovaries in females and the testes in males. The main two are luteinizing hormone (LH) and follicle-stimulating hormone (FSH).

WHAT IT DOES The follicle-stimulating hormone, as the name suggests, stimulates the follicles in your ovaries to mature each month (follicles contain potential eggs). In men, FSH is involved in sperm production. The luteinizing hormone stimulates secretion of oestrogen and progesterone in the ovaries. It's also involved in the development of the corpus luteum – the follicle that releases the egg which closes and becomes the corpus luteum (more of which later). In men, it stimulates the secretion of testosterone in the testes.

To find out how these all interact during your monthly menstrual cycle, see the 'Problems with menstruation' section, page 76.

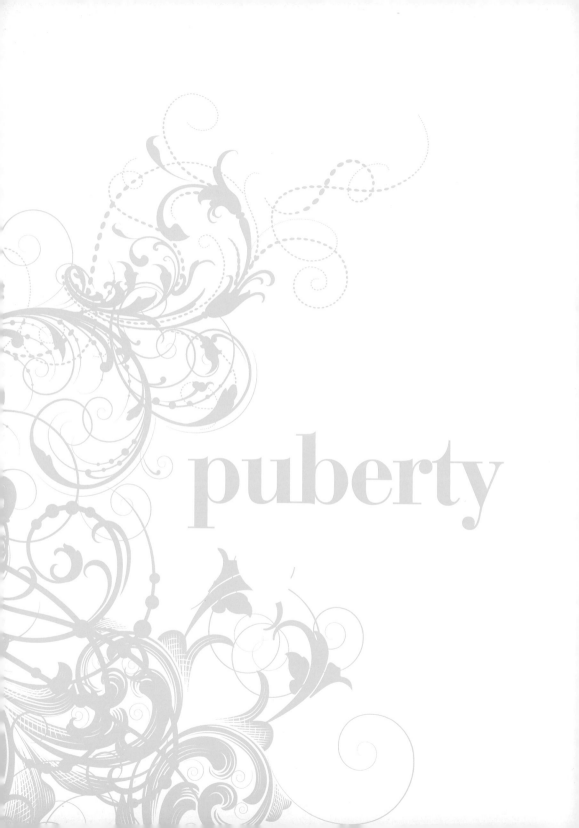

puberty

So you've hit puberty – what an exciting time! Don't believe all the negative hype about your teenage years being tough. If you're willing to put in some healthy groundwork, they can be truly wonderful. This is a time of transition, a time to be celebrated. You're becoming a woman – vibrant, intelligent, full of life and ideas and enthusiasm.

Your health, diet and lifestyle as a teenager lay the foundations for how healthy you are later in life. The habits you form over the coming years will stay with you – so I'm here to make sure those habits are positive, empowering ones.

While we're all born with certain traits or genetic susceptibilities, we can also make choices to give ourselves the best possible future, in terms of our wellbeing. It's worth adopting a diet and lifestyle now that will help to build strong bones, feed your brain, produce great skin and give you a good balance of fat and muscle in your body.

Now there's no denying it can be easy to fall into less positive habits as a teen. Whether it's poor eating, giving up on exercise, letting your moods rule you or falling prey to peer pressure and addictive behaviours you'll later regret (and, trust me, you will regret them), I've seen it all. For example, I'm amazed at how little some teenagers eat. Many drink no water. Several girls I've come in contact with often leave the house with no breakfast and eat very little until their evening meal. What they do eat tends to be rubbish.

But I'm not about to chastise you. You have my sympathy for how tricky finding a fun balance between healthy living and new-found freedom can be. Puberty can be difficult at times. Your body is releasing a cocktail of hormones that, if not kept in check, conspire to affect your emotions, your looks and your energy levels. Sometimes it's a struggle to get out of bed – let alone make all the right food and lifestyle choices when you do so (*and* be nice to your mum!).

So I'm not going to give you a prescription for what to eat at every meal or how to live each day. But I am going to point out the most important aspects of your health as a growing woman, and the areas you can't afford to neglect.

'Remember, part of becoming a grown up means taking responsibility for your own choices. So why not choose to feel amazing?'

What *is* puberty, exactly?

Puberty marks the beginning of your fertile, reproductive years. In girls, it usually happens between the ages of ten to sixteen (a couple of years later for boys). It's accompanied by a large increase in the production of female hormones and physical and emotional changes that take you into womanhood.

When puberty begins, your brain releases a hormone called gonadotrophin-releasing hormone (GnRH). This triggers the pituitary gland to release luteinizing hormone (LH) and follicle-stimulating hormone (FSH). In boys these hormones trigger the production of testosterone and sperm in the testes. In girls these hormones stimulate the ovaries to produce oestrogen and progesterone. It is largely the increase in oestrogen, progesterone, FSH and LH that causes the physical changes in a girl's body during puberty. Periods usually start between two and two and a half years after a girl's breasts start to develop. The onset of periods is called the menarche.

One thing you'll almost certainly notice is you'll get taller and fill out. Lots of girls have a growth spurt during puberty, usually before their periods start. It's not unusual to grow a few inches in height over a year. The rise in the female hormones, oestrogen and progesterone, also leads to changes in body shape, with your hips getting wider in proportion to your waist, and your breasts developing (for more on this, see 'Breast tenderness', page 69). It is normal for girls to gain some weight at this time. So don't freak out about it.

You'll notice hair starting to grow around your genitals and under your arms – usually after the breasts have started forming. This hair is fine to begin with, thickening and becoming curlier as puberty goes on. If you haven't already, you'll also develop hair on your legs and arms. This is all completely normal. Your mum, older sister or another relative can show you different ways to remove unwanted hair on your legs or under your arms.

The other major change, of course, is menstruation – your monthly bleed or period – which starts in puberty and continues until the menopause, around the age of fifty-one. The average age for a first period is twelve and a half, but everyone's different. You're likely to start yours around a similar time that your mum did. It's worth keeping some sanitary protection at home or in your school bag so you're ready. Sanitary towels are easiest at first, but some of you may want to start using tampons after a while. Your mum, sister or friends can advise. You can read more about periods on page 76.

All this change might sound scary but it's perfectly natural and something to be celebrated, rather than feared. And you won't be surprised to read that a decent diet and regular exercise will make all these transitions much smoother and easier to deal with.

The importance of good nutrition

The food habits you get into now will lay down the foundations for the future health of your body. I'm talking skin, bones, reproductive health and organ development. Every mouthful counts! I can't emphasize this enough – after all, it's what I'm all about. Now more than ever is the time to start making positive food choices. What you do now lays down the healthy foundations within your body for the future – bone health, skin, organ development, reproductive health. These are things that may not be in the forefront of your mind as a teenager but good habits now will reap rewards over a lifetime.

A teenage girl grows faster during adolescence than at any other time in her life, save for infancy. That requires a mountain of vitamins and minerals best found in food, as well as an average of 2,200 calories a day. Bear the following in mind and you'll sail through puberty, bursting with health.

Top foods for puberty

ESSENTIAL FATS The omega-3 and omega-6 essential fatty acids are so-called because they are vital for hormone, skin, nail and hair health, energy, brain function and cardiovascular health. They are found in oily fish, shelled hemp seeds, pumpkin seeds, sunflower seeds, flaxseeds and walnuts as well as the cold pressed oils of these nuts and seeds. Eat them every day.

FRUIT AND VEG Eat five to eight portions of fruit and veg a day. I know everyone talks about getting your 'five-a-day' but really this should be a bare minimum – I'd love you to eat more, please. A diet high in fruit and vegetables will make you less susceptible to many diseases, because they're bursting with vitamins, minerals, fibre and other important nutrients called antioxidants (which offer protection against many conditions of ageing).

> **GREENS** Make sure your quota includes plenty of green stuffs! Green vegetables provide calcium, magnesium and B vitamins that are vital for female hormone balance as well as blood-sugar balance and energy.

> **VEGGIE MEALS** Have some vegetarian meals each week – animal protein is often high in saturated fat, is hard to digest and often constipating and, in excess, increases your risk of developing many illnesses later on. I am not saying that you should not eat meat but do vary your diet, eating more than just meat. You just need to make sure your veggie meals contain protein, so include beans, pulses, quinoa, soya, eggs or cheese.

> **WHOLE GRAINS** Choose these rather than white, refined foods – they are *way* richer in fibre and nutrients than their refined counterparts. Fibre is important for hormone health, digestive health, blood-sugar balance, cardiovascular health, and makes you feel fuller so you're less likely to overeat.

> **WATER** Drink six to eight glasses of water or herbal tea a day – hydration is important for all aspects of health, both now and the future. This is a good habit to get into.

> **IRON** One study found that even a mild iron deficiency can result when menstruation kicks in and your diet is poor. Another study resulted in lower test scores in maths.

BREAKFAST All the meals you eat in the day are important but breakfast is *key*. Eating first thing in the morning benefits thinking power and helps to maintain a healthy body weight. It'll boost your concentration at school or college and make you less likely to reach for sweets and chocolate at break time. A healthy breakfast containing complex carbohydrates can set you up for stable blood-sugar levels, steady energy and clear concentration over the day, as opposed to the blood-sugar roller coaster that kicks in with a sugary breakfast, or no breakfast at all.

Types of iron

There are two types of dietary iron: haeme iron from animal products and non-haeme iron from plant sources. Haeme iron is generally more easily absorbed than non-haeme iron. However, the absorption of non-haeme iron is increased by consuming vitamin-C-rich foods with the iron-rich plant foods. Sources of haeme iron include: meat, eggs, fish and poultry. Sources of non-haeme iron include almonds, figs, dulse, kelp, kombu, wakame, parsley, watercress, broccoli, kale, quinoa, amaranth, oats, lentils, millet, rye, prunes and nettles. Consume these foods with vitamin-C-rich fruit and vegetables such as broccoli, lemons, tomatoes, peas, sweet potatoes, peppers, berries, kiwi fruits and blackcurrants, A good iron-rich breakfast would be porridge with prunes and berries. An iron-rich lunch or dinner could consist of chicken or fish with sweet potatoes and watercress salad.

Milk

Many people pour cow's milk on their breakfast cereal. However, some people are lactose intolerant and a cow's milk allergy has also been linked to conditions such as eczema and irritable bowel syndrome (IBS). Alternatives to cow's milk include goat's and sheep's milk or soya, rice, oat or almond milks – and some people find that boiling cow's milk first can make it easier to digest. However, it should be noted that plant-based milks do not have the same nutritional content as milk from animals. Almond milk is rich in calcium but if you do not use either this or an animal milk it is important that you include other calcium-rich foods in your diet. Good sources of calcium include green vegetables, almonds, hazelnuts, tahini, canned fish with bones and sea vegetables.

Yoghurt also tends to be easier to digest than cow's milk as it has been partially broken down by the beneficial bacteria it contains so try having yoghurt instead of milk.

Healthy breakfast ideas

Porridge with shelled hemp, flaxseeds or cinnamon

Breakfast smoothie made with fruits including avocado, flax oil and an option of soya milk

Fruit salad – follow this with another option

Rye toast with nut butter: try cashew-nut butter or almond butter instead of peanut butter for a change

Natural yoghurt with nuts and seeds

Sugar-free muesli with rice milk, almond milk or goat's milk

Herb omelette with plenty of your favourite fresh or dried herbs

Recipe for home-made muesli
Combine oat flakes, hazelnuts, sunflower seeds, pumpkin seeds, chopped Brazil nuts, goji berries, raisins and chopped apricots. Make a large container of this to use throughout the week. Soak it overnight in rice or oat milk and natural yoghurt to make it both delicious and easy to digest.

More diet tips

Eat healthy snacks – snacking can be a good way to keep your energy levels stable. However, you need to choose the right ones. Fruit, nuts, seeds, vegetable sticks and dips, olives and avocados all get my vote.

Check out your canteen. Is the food on offer there nutritious? It's tempting to order pizza or chips if it's available every day and that's what your friends choose. Consider taking a packed lunch from home to have more control. Or commit yourself to making healthier choices in the school lunch hall and don't eat the same thing day in day out.

Encourage your family to sit down together at a table to eat meals, and turn the TV off. You can inspire your parents and siblings to healthier ways, too!

Learn to cook for yourself – offer to cook for your family once or twice a week. Experiment with different foods and recipes. Work out what you like and what combinations work well together. Being able to cook gives you independence and the chance to eat well for ever.

Get into the habit of reading labels – if you read a list of ingredients and you don't know what half of them are, the chances are they are not going to do you much good. Reading the label can give you a better insight into what you are actually eating than the picture on the packet.

Find your local health-food shop – it's a good way to get on the path to healthy eating. Here you'll discover a wider range of whole grains, pulses, nuts, seeds, herbal teas and milk alternatives than in your average supermarket.

Food swaps

Don't just reach for your favourite tuck-shop snack when you're on a break at school or college; substitute it for one of my supersnacks. (OK, some of them need a little forethought and preparation at home, but I promise you'll look and feel far better for it.)

SWAP: High-sugar, low-fibre cereal with sliced white toast and sugary jam – this is high in sugar and refined carbohydrates that will upset blood-sugar levels causing highs and lows of energy, mood and concentration.
FOR: Home-made muesli and rye toast with nut butter. This is rich in fibre and complex carbohydrates that will give you steady energy and will aid concentration throughout the morning. It will also supply you with essential fats needed for brain function and hormone balance.
(See recipe for home-made muesli on page **34**)

SWAP: Garlic bread
FOR: Wholemeal bread dipped in olive oil and garlic

SWAP: Crisps
FOR: Toasted pumpkin seeds and pine nuts or make your own crisps from beets or sweet potatoes. Here's how: Preheat oven to 200°C. Thinly slice beets and sweet potatoes. Place on a tray, drizzle with some olive oil.
Bake in the oven for 45 minutes until crispy.

Also try my Crunchy Kale Crisps. My teenage clients love them: Preheat oven to 180°C. Line a baking tray with foil and brush with olive oil. Cut the kale leaves into wide slices and arrange them evenly on the baking tray. Bake for 15–20 minutes, stirring them at least twice. Season with dried herbs.

SWAP: Chips
FOR: Oven-roasted sweet potato chunks

SWAP: Chocolate mousse or trifle pot
FOR: Stewed apple or berries, with a drizzle of honey

SWAP: Chocolate bar
FOR: Fruit, nut and seed bar

SWAP: Chocolate milkshake
FOR: Cacao and yoghurt rice/almond milkshake with
a teaspoon of agave syrup (optional)
You can make it yourself: Into your blender place: 1 banana,
4 fluid ounces rice milk or almond-rice milk, 1 teaspoon agave
and two heaped tablespoons of raw cacao powder. Blend
until smooth with unsweetened natural yoghurt.

If you're a fizzy drink fan, try gradually swapping down
through the following list of drinks. You'll find that your sweet
tooth gradually disappears and you'll end up preferring the
more nutritious carrot juice!

Cola (diet or normal)
TO
Natural ginger beer
TO
Sparkling elderflower
TO
Strawberry and raspberry juice
TO
Organic carrot juice

Daily supplements during puberty

You should always do your best to eat a healthy and varied diet, but if you have a deficiency in a certain area you can take a supplement to top you up. Check with your medical doctor before taking supplements.

- Good-quality multivitamin and mineral formula
- Green superfood (such as spirulina or wheatgrass)
- Omega-3 essential fatty acids – a fish-oil or flaxseed oil supplement

The following are very useful so could be taken on rotation. For instance, take iron for a month or so until the bottle is finished and then move on to a good bone-health formula. You do not need to take them all at once.

- Iron (especially if you have heavy periods or are vegetarian). You can get nice-tasting, non-constipating, plant-based liquid iron from a health-food store.
- Zinc is absolutely essential for growth. Check your nails and see if you have any white spots. If you do, this might be a sign that you need more of the mineral zinc. You can find zinc capsules in a health-food store. This supplement may only be needed for a short period of time.
- Sublingual B12 is useful if you are vegetarian. It simply dissolves under the tongue. Find it in health-food stores.
- A good bone-health formula (see page 41).

Feed your bones

Did you know about 95 per cent of the maximum strength of your skeleton is laid down by your late teens? So feeding and protecting your bones during this major growth period is vital.

Most people achieve their maximum bone density in their twenties. After this age, bone mass starts to decline gradually. This is entirely normal. Osteoporosis can occur if bone mass declines faster than normal. This is a debilitating condition in which bones become fragile and porous, making fractures and all their associated problems more likely. Osteoporosis is not a rare condition. According to the National Osteoporosis Society, one in every two women over the age of fifty suffers a fracture due to fragile or brittle bones.

It's easy to take your skeleton for granted now while you're young, strong and mobile. But achieving maximum bone mass really will pay dividends in decades to come.

A good start is to take weight-bearing exercise at least three times a week. This doesn't necessarily mean lifting dumb-bells, just any activity in which your bones and muscles support a weight – which can be your own body weight. So running, jumping, circuit-training, netball and dancing are all weight-bearing. Swimming or cycling, for example, are not.

A word of caution: be careful using weights machines or free weights in the gym while you're still young. Always seek the advice of a gym instructor or personal trainer and keep the weights low. It's easy to damage yourself while your skeleton, muscles and ligaments are still growing.

To safeguard your skeleton, avoid:

> Smoking and drinking alcohol. These are detrimental to your health in so many ways, but they can literally leech vital bone-building nutrients from your body.

> Inactivity.

> Being underweight or anorexic.

> Fizzy drinks – the acids in these drinks need to be neutralized. Your body will take alkalizing minerals, such as calcium and magnesium, from your bones in order to do so. What scares me is the sheer number of teenagers who drink only fizzy drinks and no water.

> Coffee and caffeinated teas which also leech vital bone minerals from your body. It's just not worth addicting yourself at an early age to caffeine. I would rather you simply avoid getting into the habit in the first place.

> Sugar and refined carbohydrates – these put you at risk of developing insulin resistance which, in turn, affects calcium metabolism (how calcium is used in the body) and bone health.

> Excessive amounts of animal protein. This creates acidity in the body that needs to be neutralized by minerals from the bones.

> Salty foods, as excess sodium increases the amount of calcium you excrete in your urine.

The following nutrients are particularly important for bone health

Omega-3 essential fatty acids have been shown to have a protective effect on the bones. They're found in flaxseeds, shelled hemp seeds, pumpkin seeds, walnuts and avocados, as well as in oily fish. Or you can take a daily fish-oil supplement or borage oil and omega-3 supplements. They come in liquids and capsules.

Calcium is vital for bone health. Dairy products like natural yoghurt, kefir, goat's and sheep's milk and cheese – but not butter – and canned fish with edible bones like sardines are excellent sources of calcium. You'll find calcium in many plant sources, including tofu, soy, broccoli, savoy cabbage, kale, Brussels sprouts, chicory, pak choi, almonds, tahini, carob, dulse, figs, hazelnuts and alfalfa.

Vitamin D helps the body to absorb calcium. Your body manufactures this vitamin from the action of sunlight on the skin. While it's important to cover up and use sunscreen to avoid burning and the risk of skin cancer, it's still important to get some sun exposure without sunscreen. About fifteen minutes a day without sunscreen is enough. In summer, get your exposure in the mornings when the sun isn't so powerful. In winter, get out into the fresh air and daylight as often as possible, even if it doesn't seem sunny. If you live in a northern climate like I did while growing up, you simply do not get enough exposure to sunlight. So there may be a need to take vitamin D supplements through the winter. Calcium and Vitamin D supplements are usually recommended only to pregnant women, the elderly and some at-risk groups – women who wear burkas for example or who do not go outside much. However, if you're worried you are not getting enough or feel you are in an at-risk group – perhaps you can't get outside much – see your GP who may advise a supplement.

Other bone essentials, which work in synergy with calcium and vitamin D

Magnesium which is found in avocados, oatmeal, prunes, dark green leafies like kale, raspberries, lettuce, nuts, seeds, sea vegetables (such as kelp, nori and wakame), brown rice, aduki beans and chickpeas. Magnesium is the mineral that mobilizes calcium into the bones and teenagers simply don't get enough. So do what your granny says and darn well eat your greens. She knows what she is talking about.

Zinc which is found in fish, meats, pumpkin seeds, flax seeds, eggs, kelp, brown rice, wheat germ and tahini.

Boron which is found in almonds, carrots, apples, pears, raisins and prunes.

Vitamin K which is found in asparagus, broccoli, Brussels sprouts, cabbage, spinach, eggs, alfalfa, kelp, nettles and miso.

It's possible to buy vitamin and mineral formulations which contain all these vital bone nutrients in one. Although diet should always come first, a bone-health supplement could be very useful during puberty.

Note: It's best not to take large dosages of supplements or any supplements over prolonged periods without seeking professional advice.

Gillian's feed your bones watercress soup

My fourteen-year-old daughter can make my delicious 'Feed Your Bones' soup. If she can do it, so can you! Get Mum to help you if you need it. Tastes exceptionally delicious, too!

SERVES 2 AS A STARTER OR
LIGHT LUNCH FOLLOWED BY A LARGE SALAD
1 tbsp cold pressed sunflower oil or extra virgin olive oil
1 medium onion, peeled and finely chopped
2 sticks celery, trimmed and sliced
1 medium sweet potato (around 150g), peeled and cut
  into roughly 2cm cubes
2 garlic cloves, peeled and crushed
500ml cold water
2 tsp organic vegetable bouillon (stock) powder
1 bag (100g) fresh watercress
1 tbsp pumpkin seeds (optional)

1 Heat the oil in a medium saucepan and cook the onion and celery very gently for 5 minutes until beginning to soften. Stir in the sweet potato and garlic and cook for about a minute.

2 Pour over the water, stir in the bouillon powder and bring to the boil. Reduce the heat slightly and simmer for 12–15 minutes until potatoes are soft. Remove from the heat and stir in the watercress. Stand for 2 minutes.

3 Blend until smooth with a hand blender, or cool for 10 minutes then transfer to a liquidizer or food processor to blend.

4 Warm through gently, then ladle into deep bowls and serve sprinkled with pumpkin seeds.

Feed your brain

It makes me angry when I hear stories on the news about exams getting easier every year because I know how hard you kids work, and how much is expected of you.

What you might not realize is that your brain is an organ, too, and it needs nourishing to keep it firing. If you want to make the most of your memory, intelligence, creativity (and avoid nodding off during double maths), you need to feed your brain. I can't promise the following tips will make your homework easier – but they just might!

- Your brain thrives on essential fatty acids, antioxidants, zinc, B vitamins and good protein. You also need steady brain fuel from complex carbohydrates.

- Good brain foods include: salmon, tuna, sardines, lean white meats, tofu, eggs, avocados, spinach, peas, pulses, beans, kelp, berries, brown rice, wheat germ, whole grains, quinoa, millet, buckwheat, oats, rye, nuts and seeds.

- Do not go hungry! Always have breakfast and a healthy snack every few hours. I want six meals a day. Breakfast, snack, lunch, snack, dinner, snack.

- The best brain food of all? Water! If you're not properly hydrated, 'brain fog', sleepiness and headaches can kick in. Drink at least eight glasses of water a day and keep a bottle of water handy to sip when studying or doing exams. The amount of water you will need depends on lifestyle, too. Drink more water if you are in a warm climate, are exercising a lot or are not getting much water from the food you eat.

A good way to check you are sufficiently hydrated is to monitor the colour of your urine. It should be pale yellow. If it gets darker this may be a sign you need to drink more. The exception may be if you have taken a supplement containing B vitamins as vitamin B2 (riboflavin) turns urine bright yellow. This is a normal reaction and nothing to worry about.

Useful supplements for exam time

Eating a healthy diet and taking regular exercise are by far the best ways of ensuring you are at your best during exam time. However, sometimes herbs and supplements can help you to deal with stress or support the immune system. Below are some ideas. Do not take them all at once – that is not necessary at all. Always seek advice from your medical doctor before embarking on any supplements and check with a herbalist for the correct dosage.

RHODIOLA AND GINSENG may both aid adrenal function, help to regulate stress and energy levels and improve cognitive function and memory. Follow guidelines on the packages.

SAGE has been traditionally used to improve memory. You can drink sage tea. A couple of cups a day would be fine.

OMEGA-3 FATS such as flax oil and fish oils are essential for brain function. Suggested dose: 1,000mg of fish oil a day. Or a portion of sardines or mackerel.

VITAMIN C AND BIOFLAVONOIDS help to protect against the effects of stress and support the immune system – this is not a good time to get ill. Suggested dose: 500mg twice a day. Make sure that you eat plenty of fruits and vegetables for their vitamin C content.

MAGNESIUM relaxes the muscles and nerves. You actually function better when your body is relaxed. Suggested dose: 200–400mg a day.

B VITAMINS are needed for brain function and energy. Look for a B complex with 50mg of each.

CHROMIUM may help to keep blood-sugar levels stable. Suggested dose: 200mcg a day.

GINKGO BILOBA has a long history of use for improving circulation to the brain. Suggested dose: 20 drops twice daily.

ACETYLCHOLINE is a neurotransmitter involved in the transmission of electrical activity in the brain. It may improve memory. Lecithin contains choline which may convert to acetylcholine in the brain. You can get lecithin granules in a health-food store and sprinkle them on your salads.

CO-ENZYME Q10 is an antioxidant which helps to produce energy in our cells. It may support brain function and the immune system thus reducing the likelihood of becoming ill at this important time.

Baked salmon with spinach and leeks

You need good fats to fuel your brain. This dish will do it. As an option you can serve with sweet potatoes and broccoli on the side for their antioxidants which are needed to support the immune system and help to prevent illness.

SERVES 4, SO THE WHOLE FAMILY CAN JOIN IN
2 leeks, washed, trimmed and thinly sliced
500g fresh baby spinach leaves
4 100g organic salmon fillets
1 tbsp olive oil
2 garlic cloves, peeled and finely chopped
1 tbsp fresh grated ginger
Juice of half a lemon
Handful of coriander leaves to garnish (and eat!!)

1 Preheat oven to 200°C/gas mark 6.

2 Gently boil or steam the leeks for 5 minutes to soften.

3 Place the spinach leaves in a medium-sized baking tin and top with the leeks.

4 Mix together the oil, garlic and ginger. Liberally brush over the salmon using a pastry brush. Place the salmon on top of the spinach and leeks. Pour over the lemon juice. Cover with tin foil.

5 Place in the oven and bake for 10 minutes. Remove and allow to rest for 5 minutes.

6 Garnish with fresh coriander leaves and serve. As an option you can add some steamed sweet potatoes and broccoli on the side. These both contain antioxidants needed to support the immune system. If you have a strong immune system during exam time, there is less chance of getting sick.

Importance of maintaining a healthy weight

Before I sat down to write this part of the book, I asked my teenage daughter what aspects of health most concerned girls of her age.

'Weight and fat,' she replied, matter-of-factly. Turns out it's the only thing most of her peers worry about. This makes me really sad, because if I could just persuade you girls to think about *health*, rather than fat, you wouldn't even have to give your weight a second thought. It would take care of itself, naturally.

There's no denying it's important – essential, even – not to become overweight or obese. So many chronic health conditions are linked to excess weight and there's certainly an obesity crisis in the Western world that can't be ignored. The earlier in life you put on excessive weight, the harder you'll struggle to keep it off as an adult.

But thanks to society's celebration of stick-thin models and celebrities, our ideas of what actually constitutes a healthy weight are somewhat skewed. So let me make one thing clear. It's normal – in fact it's healthy and desirable – for teenage girls to gain some weight. Puberty is a period of intense growth and development. And while boys gain more fat on their trunks and lose it on their arms and legs during the adolescent growth spurt, you girls tend to put it on evenly all over your bodies. Women naturally have more body fat than men and you're turning into a woman.

What you need now is plenty of nutritious food to grow into your natural body weight. What you should *not* do is overeat on junk food that's lacking in nutrients *or* try to keep your weight down by denying yourself food or following crash diets or faddy eating plans. You'll become ill.

If you read in a magazine or book about a diet that claims you'll lose a lot of weight in a short amount of time, it's not healthy. Believe me. Likewise if it suggests you'll lose weight by cutting out whole food groups like complex carbs and eating just a few types of unhealthy foods. Such fad diets may lead to weight loss initially but this is usually followed by weight gain when the diet finishes or when hunger takes over.

Gillian's tips for a healthy body image

Educate yourself. The fact that you're reading this book is a fantastic start. Instead of reading about the latest 'wonder diet', read up on healthy foods, how to cook and healthy living.

Forget faddy diets, calorie counting or obsessively weighing yourself. If you simply follow the advice on healthy eating earlier in this chapter, your body will reward you.

Learn to cook – experiment with different recipes and foods. Even if you have been born into a family that has no clue about food, cooking or anything healthy, you can change the situation for yourself and it may just rub off on everybody else in the house, too. Visit a health-food shop. Cook for your family and friends. Enjoy your food and make eating an enjoyable part of your life.

Avoid sugar, refined carbohydrates, junk foods, caffeine and alcohol. These provide 'empty' calories – they're not nutritious and won't satisfy you, so you'll soon be searching the kitchen cupboards for something else.

Aim to eat small, regular meals and snacks throughout the day – three main meals and three small snacks is ideal. This will keep blood-sugar levels balanced and reduce energy slumps, cravings and overeating.

Talk to your friends and family. We all need to support each other when it comes to establishing good eating habits, a healthy attitude to food and a healthy lifestyle. Good intentions are easier if everyone is on board.

Be strong and true to yourself. Peer pressure, or even pressure from family, can lead to eating or drinking substances you would rather not put into your body and to leading a lifestyle that is not what you really want.

Celebrate diversity – we're all unique, with different body shapes and features. Some are naturally curvy, some are long-limbed, some are petite, some have bigger hips ... The variety is endless. That's the beauty of us.

Important lifestyle advice for puberty

Make exercise a habit

It seems to me that teenagers today are far less active than in years gone by. I'm not saying it's your fault – schools don't seem to offer enough PE to really keep you fit and interested. And while walking everywhere is great, sometimes it's just not safe. Then there's the homework: piles of it. When are you supposed to fit it all in? I hear you say. Organize your day so that you get some exercise. Make sure you find a fun activity you can do when you get in from school – turn on the radio and dance to your favourite music. Just go crazy and have fun.

It's easy to be put off exercise if you're not a fan of team sports or athletics. I know there are some games teachers who lose interest in pupils who don't make the netball or hockey teams. You have my full sympathy if that's you. But let's think outside the box (or the pitch) just for a minute.

Exercise doesn't have to mean competing at a sport or running round a field if that's not your thing. Keeping fit can be walking the dog, helping with the gardening, going for a bike ride. It can be going to dance classes, horse-riding, ice-skating or swimming. I must tell you that I have started hip-hop dance classes (yes, me!) and I absolutely love it. I take my teenage daughter with me, too. You get fit and have fun at the same time. You can be doing an aerobics DVD, chasing your wee brother or sister around the place, or dancing yourself dizzy at a disco. So long as you're active, the choice is yours.

And why, I hear you ask, is fitness so very important? Well, I couldn't begin to tell you how many studies there are linking lack of exercise to serious health problems in later life. Exercise helps to normalize weight, appetite and blood sugar levels. It builds a strong musculo-skeletal system. (Building strong bones in adolescence is particularly important for reducing the risk of osteoporosis later in life. Evidence suggests that healthy early life practices, including regular physical activity contribute to greater bone mineral mass and optimal peak bone mass.)

Exercise strengthens your heart, improves circulation and boosts your mood, helping you to avoid depression and making you feel more confident. If you make regular activity a habit now, you're more likely to continue with it as an adult and you'll reap the benefits throughout your life.

Try to do something for half an hour, most days a week, that gets you at least a little out of breath. Encourage your friends and family to get up off the sofa and join you, too. It won't be long before you notice you have more energy, you're sleeping better and your skin looks great. Not a bad pay-off, eh?

For the sporty: a few extra pointers

If you take part in regular sporting activities, first of all, good on you! And, second of all, you'll need to pay extra-special attention to your diet to keep yourself in peak physical condition. While exercise is absolutely a good thing, it does increase your nutrient, water and calorie needs. So remember:

1 Fuel yourself
Much of the fuel you use during exercise should come from glucose stored in the cells of the body, known as glycogen. To make sure your glycogen stores are high, eat a good range of complex carbohydrates like fruit, vegetables, brown rice, quinoa, oats, rye, barley, buckwheat, millet and pulses. If you're exercising for more than an hour, keep your blood-sugar levels topped up during your workout so you don't run out of energy. Natural sugars are better for you, so sip on diluted fruit or vegetable juices rather than energy drinks to keep your energy levels topped up.

2 Stay hydrated
When we get dehydrated our muscles don't work well, reaction times slow down, energy flags and concentration goes. Water is fine but diluted fruit and vegetable juices are sporting multi-taskers as they also provide energy. Avoid drinks containing sugar and artificial sweeteners.

3 Replenish and recover
After exercise, eat or drink something containing carbohydrates within 20 minutes of finishing. This helps to bring blood-sugar levels back to normal so you're not starving later. Drink some water or juice to rehydrate. In order to fully restore glycogen levels and to repair and rebuild muscles, eat a meal containing complex carbohydrates and protein within two hours. You've earned it!

4 Repair
During exercise your muscles and joints are put under strain. Antioxidants are the tools used by your body to reduce any damage and speed repair (so you don't ache the next day or sustain injuries). Antioxidants include nutrients such as zinc, selenium, vitamins A, C and E and lipoic acid. The best sources are fruit, vegetables, nuts and seeds (which also contain essential fatty acids needed to keep the joints well lubricated) so these are great snack choices for sportswomen!

Resist peer pressure and addictive behaviour

As you're growing up you're enjoying more freedom, more choices. You may have an allowance or a part-time job that gives you access to a little money to spend as you wish. My advice would be to avoid the temptations of sweets, crisps, fast food and fizzy drinks. They're OK from time to time, but if you make them a regular feature in your life, your health – and your looks – are going to suffer. Leave the junk to other people. If you eat junk, you'll eventually look like junk and ultimately feel like junk. Get the message?

You may also find cigarettes, alcohol and even drugs creeping onto that list of temptations. Please avoid them. They may not seem addictive at first, but we know they are. The longer they're part of your life, the harder they are to give up. Ask any adult smoker if they're glad they started and I'm willing to bet not one of them will say 'yes'. No smoker wants their child to become a smoker. You know why? Because it's emotionally and physically addictive, it costs money, it ruins your health, your skin, your teeth and it makes you smell. No one likes kissing a smoker. Trust me, the friend who thinks he or she is 'cool' because they smoke cigarettes or drink alcohol is far more insecure than you think. Having the confidence and strength of mind to say 'no thanks' shows you're more grown up than they'll be for a long time to come.

And a final word about sex. Now I'm a nutrition expert not a sex expert! So I'm not about to tell you what you should or shouldn't be doing, with whom, or when. But it wouldn't be me if I didn't say something to you, would it? SO, WAIT!! Allow yourself to be a kid as long as possible without the complications and emotional entanglements of a sexual relationship. You have your whole life ahead of you for that.

Human papillomavirus vaccine

There are many strains of the sexually transmitted human papillomavirus (HPV), a few of which are thought to cause cervical cancer (see page 132), and some of which cause genital warts (see page 156).

The HPV vaccination brand offered in schools is Cervarix. This offers prevention against the two most significant cancer-causing strains and is offered to schoolgirls aged twelve to thirteen on the NHS, with a catch-up programme being rolled out for girls up to eighteen. It is offered to young girls because it is more effective if given before sexual activity (and any possible HPV infection) begins.

You may choose to have the vaccination privately. If so, you will probably be offered a different vaccine, Gardasil. This offers protection against four types of cancer-causing strains. Be aware that you will still always need to attend your cervical screening tests. However, it's worth knowing the following:

- The vaccine does not protect against all strains of HPV that cause cancer.

- Trials have only been carried out in nine to twenty-six year-olds, so the effectiveness of the vaccine for older women is unknown.

- Adverse effects that have been reported include dizziness, nausea, headaches and rashes.

Make an informed decision about whether or not you want the vaccine and that way you will be happy with your choice. So do your research thoroughly.

I am aware that teenage hormones mean you're probably becoming interested in sex so all I'm going to say is this: be confident, respect yourself and ignore pressure to do anything except what *you* want to and feel ready for. Don't be afraid to talk honestly to friends, teachers or parents about your feelings, or to ask questions. And if you do decide to have sex, stay safe and always use a condom. But I would be a lot happier if you just focused on having a healthy body, learned to look after yourself properly when it comes to food and what to put into your body and waited until your twenties for all that sex stuff!!

And so to bed . . .

Teenagers love nothing more than a lie-in. Dragging my daughter out of bed for school can be quite a challenge, I can tell you. But then I was the same at her age. The fact is, you love your sleep because you *need* to sleep. Puberty is a period of huge physical growth and repair and most of that happens while you're tucked up under your duvet.

If you want to feel your best – alert and energized at school and not too knackered to enjoy yourself at weekends – then don't wait until Saturday morning to catch your extra zeds. Try to get to bed at a decent hour on week nights. Tempting as it is to stay up late, the more hours' sleep you can clock before midnight, the better. Otherwise you'll oversleep in the morning and you won't feel refreshed. Aim for nine hours a night (you might even need ten).

Try to build some relaxation into your week, too. We spend so much of our 'downtime' stimulated by the internet, emails, instant messaging, texting. Sometimes it's good to switch everything off and just relax. Chat to your family, listen to some chilled-out music, have a long bath or read a good book. Just 'be'.

Puberty – energy synchronization

Puberty is the time when the energy centre, a chakra called 'solar plexus', opens. This energy centre is situated above the belly button, or around the tummy region. It is associated with the colour yellow and its element is fire. You may have heard the expression 'fire in the belly'. This energy meridian, when free flowing, allows us to stand our ground on who we are, asserting your personal power: self-esteem, personality and sense of self. This region is the seat of your sensory antennae system telling us what feels right or wrong; it's where 'gut feeling' comes from, your instinctive feelings, your emotions. You need to 'listen' to this energy region to find out what you really want in life, what you actually feel is best for yourself and who you really are. If energy is flowing freely in this centre, you may experience joy and radiate happiness to those around you. A sense of peace, harmony, self-acceptance (and acceptance of others) permeates.

Teenagers with good energy flow through this area may relate better to others, have a clear sense of purpose, good self-awareness and self-confidence. They may start to develop ideas about how they want to look, what their role in life may be, what is important to them and their priorities. This energy centre tells us what feels right for ourselves, what we need to know. It is in the teenage years when this energy centre begins to take its vibrational shape.

However, during times of change and development, there may be disturbances in the energy flow. A blocked energy flow from teenage years can hang around for a lifetime.

Blockages in the solar plexus can lead to emotional problems such as low self-esteem, over-sensitivity to criticism or mood swings. You may get upset when people and things don't fit in with your needs. If there are emotional traumas (which everyone has at some point), there are greater chances of blockages in this region.

The blocked energy can create unwanted physical matter, sickness or a lack of balance physically and metaphysically. When we can synchronize our body's physical and metaphysical energies, we are then on the path to wellness on all levels, because the energies are flowing freely.

Here are some recommendations to support energy flow through the solar plexus during puberty and at any age:

LAUGH It's great for energy flow through the solar plexus.

CRY Crying is essential. Try not to suppress your tears if you feel them welling up. It is fine to have a good cry sometimes, so just go with it. You'll feel better for it. Most important is to feel your feelings. There is nothing to fear about sadness, or grief, or upset. Know that the horrible feelings will go away eventually, especially if you don't fear or resist them ('What you resist, persist.'). The sad feelings are simply a wonderful part of your learning process, one of life's gifts.

GET CREATIVE Allow your own creativity to manifest itself. Do something that resonates with your gut feeling like sculpting, painting, dancing, singing, writing, story-telling, playing a musical instrument, or whatever. But don't worry if you think you're not 'artistic'. If any of these exercises sounds fun, just do it anyway. Ask yourself, What would be fun to do? What feels good? What speaks to you? Do you get a stir in your tummy when you think about one of these creative tasks? If so, do it.

BOOGIE Physical activity is generally great for energy flow. I love free-style dancing, any dancing – hip-hop, street, jazz, ballroom – whatever turns you on! Yoga and chi gung are particularly helpful as well as dancing, hula-hooping, aerobics, stretching, trampolining, skipping, walking, climbing and anything else that takes your fancy.

FOODS Foods to support this energy centre include millet, short-grain brown rice, quinoa, flaxseeds, ginger, lemon balm, turmeric, cumin, cinnamon, saffron and fennel.

OILS Helpful essential oils include rose, neroli, frankincense, ylang ylang, myrrh and lemon balm (melissa). Combine four drops of one or more of these oils with two teaspoons of almond oil and massage into the abdomen, between your lower ribs and your belly button.

Quiet time

In order to learn awareness of this energy centre and to notice the real you, you need quiet time. Please spend a few minutes in the morning and/or at night doing the following energy exercise for free flow of the solar plexus:

1   Sit in a chair or lie down comfortably. Listen to your breathing for a minute. Imagine that the oxygen is filling up your whole body from the legs, tummy, back, chest, arms, neck and head. As you exhale, imagine that you see the air leave your body. And just listen to the inhalations and the exhalations. You need not do anything as you are simply noticing this process and listening to the peace of your own breath. That's it.

2   Then place your hands palms down towards your tummy, just on top of and above your belly-button. With your hands, simply feel your tummy region and just be and continue

to listen to your breathing. All you are doing is feeling your tummy region with your hands and relaxing for another minute – noticing, listening – nothing else.

3   Continue to feel the sensation of your tummy region with your hands. Now imagine that you can see inside your tummy or that you are actually able to travel inside that region of your body. What do you see inside? What do you feel? What do you notice? What does it look like? Pretend that you are a student of your own body in life school rather than high school. For about one further minute simply take note, a mental note, of what you are noticing. This is your study.

4   Now visualize a beautiful vibrant white or (yellow) light of energy swirling around inside your tummy region. You can then imagine that the yellow energy grows as it swirls throughout your body and envelops the whole room or the whole world.

5   Finish by noticing and listening to your breathing. Spend less than a minute to be with your breathing and feel and notice your whole body. Just be.

This energy flowing exercise is now complete. Please do it each day – it shouldn't take you more than four or five minutes. You are making a deeper physical and metaphysical connection with your solar plexus and with your whole self.

Gillian's personal note to teenagers
Remember, you need to be your own person. When you make lifestyle changes, you may worry that people around you are making judgements about you and your behaviour. Explain why you are taking such positive steps, what works for you and why you do it – you never know, friends and family might decide to make some healthy life changes themselves.

Puberty – common conditions

Acne

Spots, zits, blemishes, pimples . . . call them what you like, they're a common feature of many teenagers' lives. Puberty hormones make your sebaceous (oil-producing) glands more active, so the skin on your face – and often your back and chest, too – can feel more greasy. Your hair may start to feel greasier as well. We all get spots from time to time, but when they become a persistent problem, we use the term acne to describe them. Acne can be anything from blackheads and red pimples to pus-filled white-heads, reddened pores and even cysts. As tempting as it is to squeeze the spots to try to remove the grease, you'll only make them redder and more noticeable, as well as risking further infection and spreading of the acne. If you continue to prod and pick your skin you could end up with scarred skin and pock marks.

What you can do

Puberty and acne do *not* have to go hand in hand. Let me assure you there's plenty you can do to keep your hormones balanced and stop those sebaceous glands from going into overproduction. Diet and lifestyle factors can contribute to acne throughout life, so by getting these sorted now, you stand every chance of having clear, healthy skin at every age.

Gillian's diet tips

Although acne is caused by underlying factors that usually correct themselves as you get older, a healthy diet will give you and your skin the best chance to resist it. I have seen immense improvements in skin tone and appearance in my own clients with a change of diet.

- Eat vegetables or salads every day with your lunch and dinner. Green leafy vegetables, carrots, onions and garlic are particularly beneficial for skin health. Include vegetable crudités in your lunch box with a dip such as hummous or guacamole.

- If you have a juicer in your kitchen, get into juicing! Good ingredients to include are carrots, lettuce, watercress, celery and beetroot. I know it sounds weird but they're really, truly tasty. If you want to sweeten the juice, add an apple to the mix. Try to drink a glass of fresh vegetable juice every day; fresh juices are so cleansing and nourishing – your skin will really thank you.

- Whole grains, such as brown rice, millet, oats, wheat germ, barley and quinoa contain magnesium and B vitamins that will help to keep your hormone levels in check. They are also rich in fibre which keeps your bowels moving. You are unlikely to have glowing skin if your bowels are congested.

- Essential omega-3 fats are vital for skin health as well as hormonal balance. So snack on sunflower seeds, raw shelled hemp seeds, pumpkin seeds and flaxseeds and aim for two to three portions of oily fish a week.

- Pumpkin seeds are an excellent source of omega-3 fats as well as the mineral zinc, another skin and hormone helper. Sprinkle a couple of tablespoons a day onto cereal or salads or just snack on them as an alternative to crisps or sweets (they're delicious lightly toasted).

- Vitamin A is also needed for healthy skin (which is why it's an ingredient in many fancy skin creams), largely due to its antioxidant properties. Vitamin A is often low in those with acne and supplementing with vitamin A may help to reduce outbreaks of acne and acne scarring. (Not to be taken by pregnant women.) It's found in a form called retinol in animal products such as eggs and oily fish like mackerel and herrings. Plus your body can make it from a nutrient called beta-carotene found in some plants. A clue: if it's orange, it probably contains beta-carotene, so seek out carrots, apricots, pumpkin and squash. Spinach and watercress are also good sources.

- Avoid fatty foods, fried foods and processed meats – these contain saturated and damaged fats that may contribute to congested pores, inflammation and hormonal imbalances.

- Likewise refined carbohydrates and sugary foods such as white rice, white bread, white pasta, pastry, cakes, biscuits, sweets, chocolate and soft drinks. These all upset blood-sugar levels which in turn can upset hormonal balance. They also feed the bad bacteria in the skin and gut that may contribute to poor skin health.

- Many people find dairy products cause skin sensitivity. They may also congest the colon and increase inflammation, so try eliminating them and see if your acne improves. Wheat and chocolate are also common culprits.

- Alcohol leeches nutrients from your body, causes dehydration and increases your toxic load by overloading your liver. So if you want to avoid acne, avoid alcopops (cigarettes too, unless you fancy a grey complexion and wrinkles by your twenties!).

- Make sure your bowels are moving daily. Foods such as fruit, vegetables, whole grains and flaxseeds are particularly good for bowel function and internal cleansing.

Water is also vital for keeping the bowels moving and for glowing skin. Aim to drink six to eight glasses of water a day.

Herbal teas can replace regular tea and coffee which may leech nutrients from the body. My favourites are nettle and dandelion leaf teas, which both have cleansing and nourishing effects that can help to improve skin health.

Flavour your foods with herbs and spices rather than iodized table salt which can aggravate skin problems. If you use salt, go for sea salt or rock salt instead.

Supplement and herb tips

Take just one or two at a time for a month or so – see which work best for you. Always consult your medical doctor before starting a course of supplements and check with a herbalist for the correct dosage of herbs.

Zinc can make a big difference to spots. You can obtain supplements of zinc but always check with your GP first.

Chromium can be helpful in reducing the amount of sugar in the blood. High blood-sugar levels can aggravate acne symptoms.

Beta-carotene, which is widely available in orange and green fruit and vegetables, can be converted into vitamin A in the body. Vitamin A is often helpful for those with acne.

Do **not** take Vitamin A if pregnant. Suggested dose: 4,000IU for three months.

The B vitamins have many functions in the body and deficiencies in the B vitamins can sometimes result in skin problems. Suggested dose: 50mg vitamin B complex for three months.

- Vitamin C helps to counteract inflammation. Suggested dose: 500mg twice a day for three months or as needed.

- Borage or evening primrose oil for essential fats as both contain GLA (gamma-linolenic acid) which has anti-inflammatory and healing effects. It may also help balance hormones if the acne is hormonal in origin. Suggested dose: 300mg of GLA equivalent for three months or as needed.

- Acidophilus with bifidus – 'friendly' bacteria – which promotes colon health and toxin elimination. Take morning and evening for a month at a time.

- The herbs echinacea, dandelion, yellow dock, burdock root and red clover are all powerful internal cleansers. Consult a herbalist who will recommend the correct dosage for you.

- The herb vitex agnus castus can help to balance female hormones if the acne seems to be linked to your cycle.

- Blue-green algae and spirulina are skin superfoods that provide beta-carotene and essential minerals. Chuck a teaspoonful into smoothies and you won't even taste them.

Skincare solutions

When your skin is greasy and spotty, it's tempting to wash it all the time using harsh, chemical products that claim to banish acne. Try to resist this temptation. Acne is inflammation so you need to give your skin some TLC – not rough it up! And, ironically, by stripping skin of *all* its oils, you may just be encouraging it to produce more, thereby worsening the problem. Try the following gentle skincare tips, instead:

- Make a natural face mask using rice milk, oats and a squeeze of lemon juice. Oats are very soothing to the skin and lemon juice has anti-bacterial and astringent properties (meaning it closes the pores).

- A combination of tea tree and camomile essential oils (two drops of each in a bowl of water) can provide a soothing, antibacterial wash.

- Look for a body wash that contains tea tree or lavender oils if you're prone to body acne.

- Clay masks, from health stores, can also be effective.

- Do *not* pick or squeeze spots! This can spread the infection and lead to scarring. Instead, dab on a little witch hazel (from chemists or health stores) using a cotton bud to reduce infection and speed healing. You can also use witch hazel all over your face, back or chest as a toner.

- Your GP can make an assessment of your skin and discuss your treatment options which might include prescribing a gentle vitamin A cream or gel. This can help to improve the appearance of acne.

- Fresh air, daylight and exercise are essential for healthy skin.

- Make-up clogs the skin so try not to wear it every day and always remove it before bed.

- Wear clothes made from breathable, natural fabrics like cotton if you're prone to body acne.

- Dry skin body brushing is great for getting your lymphatic system moving and improving toxin elimination via the skin. Sweep a natural-bristle brush all over your body (except your face), before your bath or shower.

Avoid touching the acne as much as possible. This tends to spread the infection. Always wash your hands before touching your face.

Do not underestimate the effect that junk food can have on your health. Your face will thank you for feeding your body well!

Anorexia nervosa

The term anorexic is used to describe someone who denies themselves food, even if they're hungry. Sufferers have an irrational fear of body fat and weight gain, and a very distorted body image.

Signs of anorexia, apart from the obvious significant weight loss (15 to 20 per cent below healthy weight), include eating only foods known to be low in calories, secretive behaviour around food and avoidance of social gatherings or meals with others present. Anorexics may also exercise obsessively and favour baggy, figure-hiding clothes. The consequences of not eating healthily will soon show with failing health, regular illnesses, missed periods and white spots on the nails (this might indicate a lack of zinc if there has been no trauma to the nail).

What you can do

If you suspect you, or someone you know, has anorexia, please do not suffer in silence. There is plenty of help out there if you ask, so seek the advice of your GP immediately. Contact B-eat for advice and support. www.b-eat.co.uk.

Body odour

Puberty is a time when you may notice that your body smells more strongly than it used to. Again, it's hormones that are the cause, encouraging your sweat-producing glands to go into overdrive. You may find you perspire more under your arms, and perhaps elsewhere on your body such as your feet, the genital region or all over when you exercise. Sweat alone isn't a problem – it's a natural mechanism by which your body cools itself down. But when it lingers on skin it can start to smell unpleasant. That's because bacteria that live naturally on the skin start to feed on it and break it down. This causes an unpleasant smell – body odour, or 'BO'.

What you can do

Take regular baths or showers and refresh areas like your armpits with a flannel if you need to. This is probably more often than you've previously washed, but it'll help to keep you clean and smelling fresh. Use natural soaps and shower products to avoid irritating the skin.

Always shower after exercise. Fresh sweat is odourless – it's when it stays on your body that it starts to whiff.

Use a natural deodorant, one that is free of aluminium – you'll find a wealth of options available in your health store. Avoid anti-perspirants as these work by blocking your pores to stop you sweating. Sweating is a form of toxin elimination so we shouldn't stop it.

Put on fresh clothes. It might sound obvious, but it doesn't matter how clean you are if the clothes you put on after showering aren't. Wash your games kit after playing sport – bacteria can survive in damp clothing and cause it to smell.

Wash your feet and change your socks regularly and avoid wearing the same pair of trainers day in, day out. Wear cotton socks and open-toed sandals or flip-flops when you can, and go barefoot at home.

Certain foods can affect how your sweat smells. For example, research has found people who consume a lot of red meat have less attractive body odour than those who don't. So if you have a body odour issue, don't overdo the red meat. Choose white meats like chicken, fish and turkey. Although garlic and spices are very good for you, their smell can come out through your sweat. Perhaps avoid a strong curry the day before an important event, like your prom!

Make sure you get at least your five-a-day of fruit and vegetables a day. They'll keep your body nourished, your bowels moving. They have what I call a quick transit time, which means they digest fairly quickly and don't hang around inside your body too long. Whole grains contain the fibre needed to keep your bowels moving. Having clogged up bowels can increase your toxic load

Water helps to detoxify the body. The cleaner you are on the inside the nicer you'll smell on the outside. So drink at least eight glasses a day.

The herb sage can help to balance excessive sweating. Suggested dose: 15 drops in water two to three times daily. You can drink sage tea too. It actually has a pleasant taste.

If you sweat copiously and can't seem to control it, see your GP. A small percentage of people have a condition called hyperhidrosis which causes excessive sweating.

Breast tenderness

Breasts usually start to grow at the beginning of puberty. This can be as young as seven or eight in some girls, while for others the growth may not begin until they're well into their teens. It's caused by an increase in the amount of oestrogen and progesterone in circulation.

Initially the growth is called budding, as small mounds appear under the nipples and areola (the dark area around your nipples). The areola may darken further as puberty progresses. Sometimes one breast starts growing before the other. This is perfectly normal.

Many girls and women have one breast larger than the other. It may change as you get older or you may always have one breast slightly bigger than the other. I remember when I was a teen, I was so worried about the left boob being ever so slightly bigger than the right that my mum eventually took me to the doctor to have it checked out. Nothing to worry about, of course. This is normal and not unusual. If breasts develop rapidly, stretch marks may appear but these usually fade over time. As puberty goes on you may get a small amount of hair growing around the areola. It's good to get into the habit of checking your breasts, so you know your body well. Don't hesitate to seek advice from your GP if you have concerns.

The breasts and nipples can be quite sore and tender when they're growing, particularly at the budding stage. This usually diminishes with time. Breast tenderness is also a common symptom of pre-menstrual syndrome (PMS) (see page 78).

What you can do

Be aware that your breasts are extra sensitive while they're growing – you may need to avoid things like contact sports, so you don't knock them. Getting fitted for a bra will also help to ease discomfort.

A healthy diet rich in zinc, essential fatty acids, vitamin E and B vitamins may be helpful for easing breast pain. Zinc is found in pumpkin seeds, eggs, fish, brown rice, wheat germ, pulses, sesame seeds, tahini and chicken. Essential fatty acids are found in hemp seeds, flaxseeds, pumpkin seeds, sunflower seeds, oily fish and avocados. B vitamins are found in eggs, spinach, fish, poultry, green vegetables, sunflower seeds, brown rice and bananas.

Bulimia nervosa

Bulimia is characterized by episodes of binge eating followed by purging – sufferers either abuse laxatives, starve themselves or make themselves sick to try to make up for excessive calorie intake. They may also exercise vigorously to burn off the calories. The binge-purge cycle is usually done in secret and can go on for years without anyone noticing, because a bulimic's weight often remains the same.

Although the secretive behaviour makes bulimia hard to spot, the health consequences are evidence. Sufferers may have swollen salivary glands, dental erosion, a frequent sore throat and ulcers, thanks to the abnormal vomiting and the acid it contains. They may also suffer dehydration, blood-sugar imbalances, an erratic heart beat, absent or disrupted periods, hair loss, premature ageing, low blood pressure, mineral imbalances, rectal bleeding and physical weakness.

What you can do

If you're bulimic (or you suspect someone you care about is), seek advice from your GP immediately. Contact B-eat for advice and support. www.b-eat.co.uk.

Glandular fever

If you have had or you suspect you have glandular fever, then you have my every sympathy. I came down with this when I was seventeen and, boy, does it make you feel *lousy*!

Glandular fever is an infection caused by the Epstein-Barr virus. Although it can occur in adults, it's most common in adolescence. You might hear it called the 'kissing disease', because the infection is passed through saliva. The virus affects your blood, glands, lymph nodes, spleen and liver.

Symptoms include a high fever, sore throat, swollen glands, headache, loss of appetite, weight loss, muscle aches and debilitating fatigue. They usually last a couple of weeks but can persist for longer, especially if you overexert yourself.

What you can do

Your GP will usually diagnose glandular fever via a blood test. However, because it's a virus, antibiotics won't work, so they'll probably only suggest painkillers to ease aches and bring down your fever. The key to recovery is rest. Don't try to do too much, too soon. You'll also need to strengthen your blood, liver function and immunity. Avoid contact with others during the feverish stage, which is the most contagious. Crucially, avoid alcohol as you may have an inflamed liver caused by the virus.

Immune-supportive nutrients

• Beta-carotene (which converts to vitamin A in the body) found in: peaches, apricots, nectarines, carrots, parsley, spinach, squash and pumpkin.

• Vitamin C found in: strawberries, blackcurrants, lemons, grapefruit, kiwi fruit, kale and goji berries.

• Vitamin E found in: avocados, olives, olive oil, cold-pressed sesame oil and wheatgerm.

• Folic acid found in: broccoli, cabbage, kale, Brussels sprouts and broccoli sprouts.

• Zinc found in: pumpkin seeds, fish, kelp, brown rice, wheat germ, beans, lentils, tahini and chicken.

• Selenium found in: Brazil nuts, herrings, sardines, chicken, dulse, garlic, kelp and wheatgerm.

• Avoid sugar, sweetened soft and fizzy drinks and overly processed foods – they're low on nourishment at a time when you need it most.

• Avoid alcohol as you may have an inflamed liver caused by the virus.

• Drink aloe vera juice before meals to support good digestion.

• Oregano, leeks, onions, garlic and chives all have antiviral properties.

• Drink plenty of fluids to avoid dehydration.

• Buy some blue-green algae (from health-food stores) and mix it into your smoothies for a super-nutrient hit.

• The herbs milk thistle and astragalus are absolute musts for liver function and strengthening immunity. Buy them in capsule or tincture form. (Check with a herbalist for the correct dosage.) You must nourish the liver. A lot of kids find that their eyesight suffers after a bout of glandular liver. That's because there is a link between liver health and the eyes. So please take heed here.

• Glandular fever can really weaken your body for the future so now is the time to do your utmost to support your entire system in every way possible. When your glands are infected, vitamin C can help so it's worth taking a supplement in powdered form and mixing it into water or juice.

• Drink nettle tea, for a mineral and energy boost, and pau d'arco tea, thought to help clear the dampness from the body that's characteristic of glandular fever.

• Taken at night, supplements of reishi mushroom, co-enzyme Q10, acidophilus and triphala powders are believed to help your liver do its job of removing toxins from the body. Check with a herbalist for the correct dosage.

Gillian's diet and supplement tips

- You'll probably feel weak and not have much of an appetite, but good nourishment is vital. Vegetable juices and soups and fruit smoothies are nutrient-rich and immunity-boosting, and easy on your digestion.

- If you have a very bad case, it is worth asking your GP to refer you to a physician who can administer vitamin C and other vitamins intravenously. Evidence for the vitamin injections is still very limited but some integrative medical clinics carry out this type of procedure. I have seen it make an enormous difference to the sufferer and speed recovery.

- You'll also need magnesium (in nuts, fish, eggs and whole grains), B vitamins (whole grains, pulses, green leafy vegetables) and the essential fats (oily fish, nuts and seeds, avocados) for healthy adrenal glands.

- You must support your immune system as it will be compromised during this time. Nutrients needed for the immune system include vitamins A, C, E, folic acid, zinc and selenium. (See box.)

'What you do now lays down healthy foundations within your body for the future.'

Mood swings

All too often, teenagers are stereotyped as moody and emotionally volatile. As if puberty doesn't put enough strain on you, now you have to put up with people criticizing your moods, decisions and behaviour, too!

The fact is, you *are* likely to feel more up and down. Not only are your hormones running amok and exerting control over your emotions, you're also growing from a girl into a young woman. During your teenage years and early twenties your brain will undergo a period of reorganization that will ultimately help you to understand your own feelings and those of others, as well as improving decision-making and self-awareness. It's a time of immense change – and who wouldn't be a bit 'weirded out' by that (as my daughter might say), every so often? You may feel more sensitive to criticism, irritable, angry and upset. You may also start to feel more strongly about what you wear, what you eat, your friends, what music you like and what you believe in. You might be talking quite calmly one minute and start snapping the next.

The good news is that puberty doesn't have to be one long emotional rollercoaster. There's lots you can do to keep your feelings on a more even keel.

What you can do

You're not alone; all adults were teenagers once, so talk to people. Sharing how you feel and what's stressing you out can help to get life in perspective. There are some things you may want to talk to your friends about, while there may be other things you would rather talk to your parents, siblings, other relatives or even your teachers about. Just knowing others understand or have been through something similar can make everything seem far less traumatic.

One of the most important factors in how emotionally volatile you are is the stability of your blood-sugar levels. A steady supply of sugar (glucose) to the brain and body helps to keep your energy, moods and emotions even. But don't think that's a green light to head for the sweet shop!

Paradoxically, one of the *worst* things you can do to keep blood-sugar levels stable is to eat sugar, as this tends to raise blood sugar rapidly and dramatically, followed by a slump when you may feel moody, angry and irritable. Physical activity helps improve blood-sugar control and your mood. Playing sports or going to the gym is great but you could just go for a brisk walk, a swim, cycle ride or dance around to the radio every day – whatever you enjoy.

See also my section on PMS (page 78) if you feel your moods worsen in the run-up to your period.

Gillian's diet and supplement tips

> Eat small, regular meals and snacks – don't let yourself get hungry. Many emotional outbursts in both adults and children could be avoided if blood-sugar levels were prevented from going too low. Eating five to six small meals or snacks over the day keeps levels and moods balanced.

> Choose complex carbohydrates as these break down into glucose slowly in the digestive tract, giving you a steady trickle into the blood stream. Complex carbohydrates are found in brown rice, oats, quinoa, rye bread, lentils and beans.

> Caffeine, alcohol and nicotine are stimulants that create a high followed by a low in which your mood can take a turn for the worse and you start to crave another pick-me-up. So just say no!

Problems with menstruation

Let's get one thing clear: menstruation itself – having monthly periods – is not an ailment. It's a completely natural and healthy feature of your reproductive years, which begin at puberty and go on until the menopause. However, the monthly cycle can throw up some problems, usually as a result of hormone imbalance, so I shall discuss those here. But, first, let's remind ourselves of some basic biology.

Usually, periods start about two to three years after you begin developing breasts. The average age is between twelve and thirteen, but they may start before or after this.

You have two ovaries, each containing thousands of follicles. Each of these follicles can potentially produce an egg that could go on to develop into a baby. However, the vast majority of them won't! The hormonal changes that occur during puberty lead to the ripening of your ovaries.

At the start of each menstrual cycle the pituitary gland in your brain releases the follicle-stimulating hormone (FSH) which stimulates one or sometimes more of the follicles in your ovaries to grow. Usually only one follicle reaches maturity each month. This is the follicular phase of the menstrual cycle. The cells around the maturing follicle produce the hormone oestrogen. This causes the lining of the uterus (womb) to thicken in preparation for a fertilized egg. This thickened lining is called the endometrium.

After about two weeks (although this varies), the rising oestrogen level in the blood signals to the pituitary gland that the egg is ready to be released. The pituitary gland then stops producing FSH and starts sending out luteinizing hormone (LH). This marks the beginning of the luteal phase, which usually lasts between twelve and fourteen days. LH stimulates the ovary to release the egg. The egg travels down one of your Fallopian tubes to the uterus. This is called ovulation. The follicular cells that remain in the ovary are now called the corpus luteum. This produces the hormone progesterone.

If the egg is not fertilized, the corpus luteum stops producing progesterone and gets reabsorbed into the ovary. The levels of oestrogen and progesterone fall and the thickened lining of the uterus starts to break up. The unfertilized egg and the lining of the uterus are eliminated from your body via your vagina. This is your period. The cycle then starts all over again.

The menstrual cycle varies in length from twenty-five to thirty-two days. Periods last from three to ten days.

A note from Gillian

Although you only suffer symptoms of PMS or other period problems for certain days or weeks of the month – and some months you may not suffer at all – my following recommendations should be adhered to *all* the time. What we're trying to do is keep your hormone levels balanced, not just reacting when symptoms present themselves. These are habits to get into for life.

Premenstrual syndrome

PREMENSTRUAL SYNDROME (PMS) is the term used to describe a wide range of symptoms that can occur in the two weeks leading up to your period. In fact, over 150 symptoms have been identified, and they may include acne, abdominal bloating, cravings, sore breasts, headaches or migraines, disrupted sleep, constipation or diarrhoea, feeling faint or nauseous, mood swings and fatigue. The key to identifying an ailment as a symptom of PMS (rather than something else) is that it will cease as soon as your period starts. There are so many symptoms and not all women will experience all – or indeed any – of them. You may also find that symptoms vary from month to month.

PMS can often seem more of a problem during puberty, as it takes time for the hormones involved in the menstrual cycle to find their natural rhythm. (In the same way PMS may seem to worsen for a few women in their forties, as the menopause approaches and hormones once again can go awry.) Changes in the brain and nervous system that happen at this time may also contribute to some of the symptoms.

What you can do

Although the symptoms may each seem very different, try to avoid treating them at a superficial level (taking painkillers for a headache, say). The real solution lies in addressing the underlying cause, which is hormone imbalance. And your diet and lifestyle can go a long way towards doing this. Stress and your emotional state can increase your chances of suffering from PMS. Learning relaxation techniques such as focusing on your breathing, listening to gentle music or meditation may all help. And don't forget exercise. It'll improve your circulation, may relieve headaches, reduce bloating and digestive symptoms and will definitely boost your mood.

Gillian's diet tips

Avoid sugary foods and refined carbohydrates. These include white rice, white pasta, white bread, cakes, pastries, sweets, chocolates and biscuits. These foods upset blood-sugar balance which, in turn, has an impact on female hormone balance. Research confirms that eating sugary foods increases PMS symptoms.

Replace refined carbohydrates with complex carbohydrates – such as brown rice, whole grain pasta, wholemeal bread, rye bread, oats and quinoa. These contain fibre which helps to keep blood-sugar levels more stable, as well as B vitamins and magnesium needed for female hormone balance.

Although you might feel like you need a pick-me-up when you have PMS, resist that coffee or cola. Consuming caffeine is associated with an increased likelihood of suffering from PMS. It's a stimulant which will exacerbate the blood-sugar highs and lows you're trying to avoid. Caffeine is found in tea, coffee, cola, chocolate and many energy drinks, as well as some over-the-counter medications including pain-relieving drugs.

Avoid drinking alcohol and smoking (including passive smoking) – both have been shown to increase PMS.

Eat nuts and seeds – the omega-3 and 6 essential fats they contain can have an anti-inflammatory effect and are also vital for the balance of your hormones and function of your nervous system. Snack on hemp seeds, sunflower seeds, pumpkin seeds, flaxseeds, walnuts, avocados and cold-pressed oils. You can also get these useful fats from oily fish such as salmon, trout, mackerel and sardines.

Eat Brussels sprouts: they may not make your hair go curly, but they can certainly improve your health in many other ways. Green vegetables, such as broccoli, kale, spinach, chard, Brussels sprouts, watercress, and chicory, are all rich in the minerals calcium and magnesium. These are both needed for hormone balance and a healthy nervous system.

If you suffer from nausea, eat small, regular meals and snacks. Keeping blood-sugar levels balanced is one of the most important aspects of reducing nausea. Always have breakfast when you get up in the morning and take healthy snacks such as fruit, nuts, seeds and vegetable crudités to school or college. And try ginger tea, made by infusing slices of ginger root in boiling water.

Gillian's supplement and herb tips

Always consult a medical doctor before taking supplements and check with a herbalist for the correct dosage of herbs.

Calcium, magnesium and vitamin D work in synergy to support hormone balance and have been proven to reduce PMS symptoms. The best way to increase your vitamin D levels is to spend time outside with some skin exposed to daylight. Just fifteen minutes in the morning sun each day is fine (don't wear sunscreen but do cover up well before you burn). Vitamin D increases your absorption of calcium.

Vitamin B6 is important for female hormone balance. The B vitamins work together and are involved in the production of energy, blood-sugar control and nervous system function. Take a B-complex supplement which includes them all.

- Vitamin B6 and magnesium work well taken together to relieve nausea.

- Vitex agnus castus is a herb which may help to control the balance of oestrogen and progesterone, and many women find it incredibly helpful in controlling their PMS symptoms.

Vanilla and cinnamon rice pudding

Brown rice is a good source of the much-needed B vitamins.

SERVES 1
350ml water or rice milk
100g organic short-grain brown rice
$\frac{1}{2}$ stick cinnamon
$\frac{1}{2}$ pod vanilla
Zest and juice of $\frac{1}{2}$ orange
1 teaspoon of agave syrup (optional)
Hulled hemp seeds

1 Place the water or rice milk in a small saucepan, add the rice, cinnamon, vanilla, zest and orange juice, and the syrup if using.

2 Bring to the boil, cover and simmer for 25–30 minutes, until the rice is cooked, stirring occasionally.

3 Sprinkle with hulled hemp seeds – a source of much-needed healthy fats.

Painful periods (Dysmenorrhoea)

Painful periods can be anything from a dull ache or dragging sensation in your lower abdomen or back to full-on cramps that make you want to take to your bed. The pain is linked to a rise in natural chemicals called prostaglandins in the body at ovulation, and usually begins just before or just after bleeding starts (therefore it's not classed as PMS). Pain can also be linked to reduced blood flow.

What you can do

With all problems related to the menstrual cycle, I'd recommend following my advice for PMS, as well as the additional tips, below. Some women find that relaxing with a hot-water bottle on their tummy or lower back offers relief. Lavender essential oil has a particularly relaxing effect. Add a few drops to a warm bath or combine three drops with a teaspoon of almond oil and massage it into your abdomen. And although you might not feel like it, gentle stretching exercises or a walk can really help.

If you are in a situation where you are missing school every month due to throwing up and terrible pain, you must see your GP. Also, in cases like this, it's worth visiting a herbalist to get a herbal formula specifically for you.

'Celebrate diversity – we're all unique. That's the beauty of us.'

Gillian's diet and supplement tips

Always consult a medical doctor before taking supplements and a herbalist for the correct dosage of herbs.

- Warm herbal teas such as chamomile, lemon balm and ginger root can help to soothe and relieve the tightness that may be causing cramps.

- Essential fats have an anti-inflammatory effect which will ease painful spasms. Take them as fish oils, flaxseed oil or GLA for maximum benefits.

- Vitamin E supplements can help to moderate levels of prostaglandins (the hormones responsible for causing the pain).

- B vitamins are essential, especially vitamin B6.

- The herbal supplement dong quai has anti-inflammatory, anti-spasmodic and pain-relieving effects.

- Cramp bark, as its name suggests, can be taken as a tincture to relieve cramps.

- Jamaican dogwood herb is helpful for severe abdominal pain.

Heavy periods (Menorrhagia)

Heavy periods – those that last for seven days or more or cannot easily be controlled with tampons or sanitary towels – are known as menorrhagia. Although annoying, this is not usually a medical problem, although in some cases it can indicate a disorder of the uterus, such as endometriosis (see page **134**). Bleeding heavily may also mean you lose a lot of iron and risk anaemia.

What you can do

If you're concerned about very heavy periods or anaemia, see your GP. I'd recommend asking your GP or natural health practitioner to check your iron levels. If they're particularly low you may need a supplement.

Gillian's diet and supplement tips

Anaemia is common in menstruating girls, especially those with menorrhagia. So eat plenty of iron-rich foods, such as eggs, fish, meat, poultry, almonds, figs, dulse, kelp, parsley, amaranth, rye, prunes, nettles, nori and lentils. Eating these in combination with vitamin C-rich foods can aid the absorption of iron. Vitamin C is found in fruit and vegetables.

Sage essential oil may help to reduce heavy bleeding. Combine two drops with a teaspoon of almond or sesame oil and massage into the abdomen during your period.

Drink nettle tea to help to raise iron levels naturally.

Irregular or absent periods

Periods can often be irregular for the first couple of years, as hormone levels adjust and your cycle establishes itself.

Irregular periods (oligomenorrhoea) usually settle down during puberty to a twenty-eight-day cycle, but if not this can indicate a hormonal problem, such as polycystic ovarian syndrome (PCOS) (see page 150). More usually it's just that your hormone levels need stabilizing through good diet and lifestyle measures. It's obviously useful to know when your period is due so you can be well prepared with sanitary protection. In later years it's also useful for family planning.

The absence of periods is known as amenorrhoea and the most common cause is pregnancy. If your periods haven't started before the age of sixteen, or if you had a normal cycle and suddenly miss three or more periods, see your doctor. Amenorrhoea can be a side effect of illness, stress, over-exercising or extreme weight loss, hence it's often seen in women with eating disorders.

What you can do

If you're concerned about irregular periods, see your medical doctor. It's essential to tackle the underlying cause and bring hormone levels into balance. You may need tests to determine if there are any medical reasons why you are experiencing problems – you may have PCOS, for example. It's important to keep a close check on your lifestyle and avoid faddy diets or extremes of exercising. If you think you may have an eating disorder, talk to your friends and parents.

See your GP for specific help and advice. I would highly recommend a visit to a herbalist, too.

Gillian's diet and supplement tips

Always consult a medical doctor and/or herbalist before taking supplements.

> The hormone-balancing herb vitex agnus castus may help to bring an irregular cycle into line or kick-start an absent one, as may dong quai.

> The herb black cohosh can help to normalize your period.

> Drinking red raspberry-leaf tea twice a day may help to tone and strengthen the uterus which can help to regulate bleeding. (This should never be drunk during the first six months of pregnancy.)

Q: Dear Gillian,

I try my hardest to be the healthiest I can be. I'm not overweight, I eat sensibly (you'd be proud!), I exercise, my skin and hair are OK. I have a good job, nice friends. My only problem is I hate what I see in the mirror. I have no confidence with the opposite sex, and I'm always cancelling nights out because I look awful. How can I feel better about myself? Charlotte, 19

A: Dear Charlotte,

There's absolutely nothing wrong with you but a chronic lack of self-esteem. So let's work on this self-image. I'll teach you how to love what you see in the mirror.

The first thing to remember is that no one will be nearly as critical about your appearance as you are.

And there is nothing more attractive than self-confidence. This does not mean being brash or arrogant, but rather exuding a quiet, inner confidence that will come through in the way you hold yourself and engage with others.

In order to feel confident from the inside out, you need to rewire your brain so that your beliefs about your appearance change. Using affirmations is a great way of changing your subconscious thoughts. Affirmations are short phrases that you repeat regularly in order to etch the thoughts onto your subconscious until they become beliefs. Here are some examples of affirmations to say out loud while looking in the mirror:

'I love myself.'
'I am beautiful.'
'I am fit.'
'I am healthy.'
'I am sexy.'
'I am confident.'

Choose three or four you like from this list or invent your own and say each of them seven times at least once a day.

Visualization is also a good way of changing the way you see yourself. This is good to do if you have a party or a night out coming up that you feel nervous about:

Sit comfortably and close your eyes. Allow your breath to flow in and out fully. Visualize yourself walking into the room with confidence. You are glowing with health and everyone is keen to come and talk to you. You take every conversation in your stride. You are confident enough to show interest in other people, to find out about them and to tell them about yourself. You feel open to opportunities.

The more you go out and experience the world and enjoy being with other people of both sexes, the less focused you will become on your appearance. You will realize that people like each other for lots of reasons, and looks have little to do with it. Show interest in other people, ask them questions, tell them about your life and experiences, hopes and dreams. Allow yourself to give and receive love – I am not specifically talking about romantic love, just love for other people generally. Feeling loved and loving is the real key to self-esteem

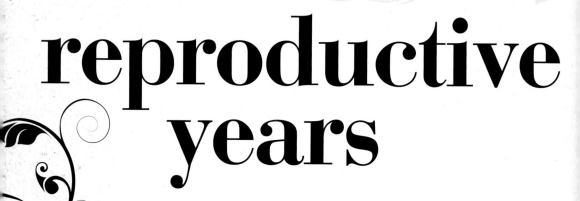

reproductive
years

Welcome to your reproductive years. In these decades, your twenties, thirties and early forties, you have the potential to be in your best physical health! Your menstrual cycle and the ups and downs of puberty have hopefully settled, and perimenopause is a long way off. In an ideal world, you'll have got into good food and exercise habits, and now know how to look after yourself. Your skin, hair and energy levels may be great. Your career may be developing, you're getting to know who you are, where your skills lie and what really interests and inspires you in life. You may be settling into a relationship, perhaps planning or raising a family. Or having children may not be for you and you've decided to pour your energies into other choices and possibilities. You'll be no less concerned about safeguarding your health and wellbeing. It's all potentially great.

But you'll notice a key word in the previous paragraph. That's right – 'potential'. I wish I could say all the clients who come to me in their reproductive years are fulfilling their health potential. Sadly, many are not. The problem is that all the choices and possibilities this life stage offer can mean you're busier than ever and have to do battle with what we call that elusive 'work-life balance'.

Managing to fit in work, a social life, relationships, family and 'me' time can be a struggle. Doing all that and shopping, preparing and eating healthy food and taking regular exercise can seem to add to the struggle (even though, believe me, it makes it much easier in the long term). If you don't get the balance right, stress and mental health issues can become a feature of this life stage. So now really is the time to learn how to put yourself first and look after your health. It can be done and you can reap the most fantastic benefits. Otherwise you'll be no good to your employer, your partner . . . and any children who might come along! If you decide you want a fit healthy life in these decades, you can have it. Plan it and make it happen. The initial dedication to planning how to get the most out of your life is worth every moment of preparation as the benefits are so many.

Which brings me nicely on to the next subject. Physically, a lot of the issues you may face at this time will involve your reproductive health. So that may be dealing with problems relating to your menstrual cycle or reproductive organs, making safe-sex choices to avoid sexually transmitted infections (STIs) and pregnancy or, conversely, trying to start a family.

The average age of first-time pregnancy in the UK is now twenty-seven and the rate of pregnancy in the thirties now exceeds that for younger women. This is not, as the media likes to portray it, always a matter of choice. Career, living arrangements, finances and available partners all play a part.

I am not going to kid you – the best time to have a baby, biologically, is between the ages of twenty and thirty-five. Fertility declines and the risk of complications increases after this age. But that's not to say it's not perfectly possible. And being an older mother has lots of advantages. You have maturity, wisdom and often money on your side and are less likely to feel you're 'missing out' because you've achieved so much in life already. But I feel I must warn you: if you want kids, do it now. Do not wait. You don't want to risk not being able to have kids at all or having no choice but to try the IVF route which may or may not work. So, please, if you want kids, go for it. What are you waiting for?

'Plan it and make it happen. The initial dedication to planning how to get the most out of your life is worth every moment of preparation as the benefits are so many.'

The importance of good nutrition

In this section, I'll talk about the best foods for fertility and pregnancy. But, of course, there's more to being a woman than bearing children (or choosing not to).

Nourishing yourself in your twenties and thirties means making sure you have enough energy and immunity to cope with the many and varied demands life can throw at you – both physically and mentally. It means doing what you can now to stave off health problems in later years – such as maximizing your bone density and avoiding becoming overweight or obese and all the related medical problems they can cause.

Top foods for your reproductive years

KELP Rich in iodine, needed for thyroid and ovarian function, kelp (seaweed) also contains many other vitamins and minerals including calcium, magnesium, iron and potassium. You can use it in so many ways: in soups, stews, casseroles and sushi.

BROCCOLI Contains a compound that helps with hormone metabolism. It's also an excellent source of magnesium and folic acid needed for reproductive health.

SHELLED HEMP SEEDS Contain a good balance of the omega-3 and omega-6 essential fats, as well as GLA – all helpful for skin, brain, hormone health and energy.

FISH A good source of protein, iron, essential fats and B vitamins, all needed for many aspects of female health.

AVOCADOS A good source of vitamin E which may help to reduce PMS symptoms as well as being full of healthy monounsaturated fats that have protective effects on the cardiovascular system, and magnesium.

WHOLE GRAINS These are rich in fibre needed for a healthy digestive tract as well as magnesium needed for a healthy nervous system, reproductive system and energy production. Try brown rice, oats, spelt, amaranth and millet.

QUINOA Also a whole grain but higher in protein than most, this is great for keeping blood-sugar and energy levels stable. Quinoa is also a good source of calcium, magnesium and B vitamins.

BRAZIL NUTS These are a top source of selenium, needed for thyroid health and reproductive health. Just three a day hits your quota!

ADUKI BEANS These are nourishing, energizing and cleansing. And fantastic if you need to keep your weight in balance. I call them my weight-loss bean.

MISO A great food for adding flavour, protein and nourishment to soups, stews and casseroles. And an easy snack, too.

RYE BREAD More filling and easier to digest than wheat bread for many people.

NETTLE TEA A good, energizing and cleansing source of iron, important during the menstrual years. Drink a couple of cups a day when you have your period.

Top snacks

Vegetable juices are a great way of upping your vegetable intake and increasing your nutrient and antioxidant levels, so get into juicing!

Apples are rich in pectin which helps to remove toxins from the body. You can put one in your bag ready for whenever you're peckish.

Almonds are an excellent source of calcium and magnesium, as well as having an alkalizing effect on the system.

Oat cakes provide a good source of complex carbohydrates for stable blood-sugar levels and sustained energy.

Dried figs are rich in iron, which is often low in menstruating women.

Pumpkin seeds are an excellent source of zinc – an essential mineral for the reproductive years. They also contain omega-3 fats, needed for female hormone balance.

Foods to avoid

- Sugar provides empty calories, leads to weight gain, increases your risk of developing diabetes (including gestational diabetes) and is associated with so many other health problems. Cakes, pastries, biscuits, chocolate, confectionery and many fast foods all contain sugar. Indulging a sweet tooth will give you a rapid energy high, inevitably followed by a sustained low – in other words, it makes you feel lousy.

- Junk foods and fast foods are high in calories and low in nutrients. They often contain additives and flavourings that have many negative effects on health.

- Alcohol generally has a negative effect on female hormone balance as well as blood-sugar balance and energy levels. And it can put you at risk of developing certain cancers later on. So watch out here!

- Artificial sweeteners are now thought to possibly upset appetite control mechanisms and so, ironically, they may ultimately feed a sweet tooth and the end result could be increased weight gain.

- Swordfish, shark and marlin may be high in mercury and other toxins which can be damaging to reproductive health and an unborn child. These are fine in small quantities.

- If you're planning to get pregnant, caffeine is best avoided as it can interfere with conception. Coffee, in particular, can upset female hormone balance and challenges the adrenal glands, creating stress and interfering with sleep.

Food swaps

SWAP: Blueberry muffin
FOR: Wholemeal fruit scone

SWAP: Cheesy pasta salad with mayo
FOR: Wholemeal pasta salad with natural yoghurt

SWAP: BLT sandwich on white bread
FOR: Bean soup with rye bread or hummous and salad wrap

SWAP: Baked potato with cheese
FOR: Baked sweet potato with ratatouille

SWAP: Chocolate chip ice cream
FOR: Frozen yoghurt

SWAP: Chocolate bar
FOR: Cacao bar

SWAP: Spaghetti Bolognese and garlic bread
FOR: Penne arrabiata with green salad

Recommended supplements

Always check with your GP before taking supplements – especially when pregnant. It is not advisable to take most supplements when pregnant.

A daily vitamin and mineral formula – suggested dose: one a day to ensure a base line of nutrition. This can be taken for three months or longer-term if you feel you need it.

Folic acid – take from the time you start trying to get pregnant up until week twelve of your pregnancy. Suggested dose: 400mcg daily if there's any possibility you might conceive.

Vitamin B complex (for energy and mood). You may not need this if you are taking a multivitamin as most multis have good amounts of B vitamins. Otherwise take as needed for energy. Do not take in the evening as this may interfere with sleep.

Calcium (the bone-building essential). Take daily alongside magnesium for bone health

Vitamin D (helps the body to process calcium). This is particularly needed during the winter months or if you do not get outside much.

Siberian ginseng (useful in times of stress). Take for three months or longer if necessary.

Agnus castus – a good, all-round female hormone balancer. Take for at least three months if needed for hormonal balance.

Feed your . . . fertility

As you get older, it may take longer to get pregnant. At the risk of repeating myself: if you really want a baby, don't wait until you have done this or achieved that! The optimum years are your twenties and early thirties for baby-making. Yes, there are women who do get pregnant later but I am telling you now, if you want to have the best chances of conceiving, get cracking on feeding your fertility and get baby-making in your optimum years.

Your GP is unlikely to do more than tell you to 'keep trying' if you report problems getting pregnant within a year. If you're over thirty-five, they will agree to investigate your fertility after six months.

I'm absolutely convinced, however, that lifestyle adjustments and optimum nutrition – for both you and your man – should be the first step in any journey towards conception. It doesn't matter if you've just started thinking about having a family, or if you've been at it for a while and are struggling and frustrated – you may never need to see that fertility doctor. The following advice will prime your body for pregnancy, and maximize your chances of natural conception.

- First of all, fat is essential to fertility. Women need body fat in order to ovulate.

- According to a study conducted by the University of Washington, if a woman's body weight is less than 85 per cent of the ideal weight there is a greater risk of infertility associated with ovulatory dysfunction. Around 6 per cent of primary infertility cases are thought to be due to being underweight.

A body mass index (BMI) of between 23 and 24 is ideal for conception. The average woman has 27 per cent of her weight as body fat. So crash diets and perpetual slimming could cause subfertility (see 'Ovulation test', page 121).

That doesn't give you a licence to eat bad food and get fat, however. Being overweight can interfere with ovulation, because the extra fat produces extra oestrogen in the system, causing an imbalance in reproductive hormones. Obesity increases the risk of infertility and losing weight has been proven to restore it in many cases.

Just as smoking when pregnant is a *bad* idea, there's good evidence that smoking when trying to become pregnant will scupper your chances. Cigarettes reduce oestrogen levels, cut the number of fertile years a woman has left to conceive, cause irregular periods and make eggs and cervical mucus less penetrable to sperm and trigger the death of egg cells. Women who *don't* smoke are twice as likely to become pregnant as women who do. Need I say more than that?

Alcohol, caffeine and stress can also be barriers to fertility. It's easier said than done but try not to get so stressed about becoming pregnant that sex becomes a function rather than a pleasure. Many couples who struggle to conceive simply aren't having enough sex because they're too stressed and tired. And several studies have shown that female orgasms are actually conducive to conception. So relax, enjoy yourselves and make this baby out of love!

Food wise, make sure you're eating at least eight portions a day of nutrient-dense fruit and vegetables; whole grains such as brown rice, buckwheat, spelt, amaranth and quinoa; and high-quality protein (from white meat, fish, eggs, nuts, tofu, sprouted seeds and legumes) at every meal. You'll also need essential fatty acids from oily fish, nuts, seeds and avocados and their oils. They have a profound effect on every system of the body, including the reproductive system, and are crucial for healthy hormone functioning.

Last but by no means least, drink plenty of water. Water plays a key role in your health. The main issue is to be heathy and avoid dehydration as the body works better when it is hydrated. If you are in good health, you increase your chances of conception.

Supplements for fertility

It is always worth consulting your medical doctor first, but I believe nutritional supplements are a fertility essential. You need iron, calcium, magnesium, zinc, vitamins A, B, C, E as well as essential fatty acids (EFAs) and probiotics. At the very least, take a good-quality, full-spectrum vitamin and mineral formula daily. All women who are trying to conceive should take 400mcg folic acid from a few months prior to trying to the twelfth week of pregnancy.

'Learn how to put yourself first and look after your health.'

Fertility foods for men

Make sure your man eats plenty of sperm-nourishing foods. So top him up with pumpkin seeds, shelled hemp seeds, mango smoothies, brown rice, oats, seaweeds (try avocado sushi), berries and cherries. Keep him off the booze, the ciggies and the white stuff (salt, sugar and bread). He will smell so much nicer, too!

My top fertility foods

Seeds

Avocados

Almonds

Figs

Berries

Pomegranates

Brown rice

Oats

Nori seaweed

Quinoa

Sprouted clover and sprouted sunflower

Turtle beans

Why not share a fertility-boosting meal with your man?

Chicken-satay-style skewers with cashew-nut dip

This tasty meal supplies zinc needed for male and female fertility.

SERVES 2
2 organic or free range boneless chicken breasts, skinned
For the marinade
Finely pared rind and juice of 2 limes
2 garlic cloves, peeled and crushed
1 tsp finely grated fresh root ginger (peel first)
1 tbsp finely chopped unsalted cashew nuts
2 tbsp extra virgin olive oil
2 tbsp chopped fresh coriander
1/2 tsp ground cumin
1/2 tsp ground coriander
For the dip
2 tbsp cashew-nut butter
2 tbsp freshly squeezed lime juice
1 tbsp finely chopped unsalted cashew nuts
1 garlic clove, peeled and crushed
1/2 tsp wheat-free tamari soy sauce
1 tbsp cold water

1 Mix marinade ingredients in a bowl. Cut the chicken into long strips and stir into the marinade. Cover and leave to marinate for 30–60 minutes in the fridge. (Soak the skewers in water to help prevent burning.)

2 Mix the ingredients for the dip in a small bowl, adding more water if necessary to make a thick sauce, and set aside.

3 Thread the chicken, a piece at a time, onto skewers.

4 Place on a rack above grill pan lined with foil and cook under a preheated hot grill for 10 minutes, turning frequently. Be careful as the sticks may be hot. Cook until lightly browned and cooked through. Serve with the cashew dip and a large salad sprinkled with raw shelled hemp seeds, steamed asparagus and baby vine tomatoes (also known as love apples!).

As a veggie alternative, try cubes of pepper, sliced courgettes and wedges of red onion. Thread onto skewers and cook as above. There is no need to marinate.

My top fertility herbs

Always check with your medical doctor or herbalist before taking a course of supplements and *stop* taking all herbs as soon as you become pregnant. Take these in rotation.

- Agnus castus
- False unicorn root
- Dong quai
- Black cohosh
- Red raspberry leaf
- Evening primrose oil
- Wild yam
- Red clover
- Liquorice root

Beware the hormone disrupters

Hormone disrupters are chemicals that may act like oestrogens in the body and mess with the action of your own hormones. Given that many of the conditions and symptoms I talk about in this book are a result of hormones being out of balance, it makes sense to avoid any nasties which could make the situation worse! Also called xeno-oestrogens, hormone disruptors often produce symptoms of too much or too little oestrogen – with potentially serious consequences for fertility and other areas of health.

Xeno-oestrogens are found in pesticides, detergents, solvents, industrial chemicals, industrial by-products, plastics, food packaging and rivers and oceans. They may get into the food chain, ending up in milk, meat, fish, animal fats, eggs, soya beans and drinking water. They are present in:

- Atrazine, a herbicide used on corn and soy crops.

- Bisphenol A (BPA), used in some plastic drinks bottles, baby bottles and in the linings of cans containing food.

- Cigarette smoke, which contains all manner of toxic chemicals, including ammonia, arsenic, benzene, formaldehyde, lead and turpentine to name but a few. This makes it highly carcinogenic (cancer-causing), especially as these chemicals are carried in the bloodstream to every cell in your body.

- Dichlorodiphenyltrichloroethane (DDT), a pesticide that has been banned but as it takes so long to break down it may still be in the environment.

- Dioxins, created as by-products of industry and incineration.

- Oral contraceptives and HRT – residues of synthetic oestrogen from these can get into the environment via our water supply. They're disrupting the reproduction of fish so what are they doing to us?

- Polybrominated biphenyl (PBBs), used as flame retardants in furniture and electrical appliances.

- Polybrominated diphenyl ethers (PBDEs), a flame-retardant found in computers, sleeping bags and now food, especially meat and poultry (which comes into contact with PBDE in the food chain and during processing or via packing materials).

- Polychlorinated biphenyls (PCBs), used in electrical equipment – these have been found to cause some birth defects and neurological impairment. They have entered the food chain and are found in fish, particularly bass and bluefin.

- Phthalates, used in plastic products, PVC, cosmetics, plastic toys and some medical instruments. They have been banned from children's toys due to their toxicity.

- Beta-hexachlorocyclohexane (Beta-HCH), a pesticide linked to the development of Parkinson's disease.

Minimize your exposure

- Avoid food and drinks wrapped in plastic as much as possible. In particular high fat foods, such as cheese, and acidic foods and drinks such as orange juice should be avoided if they are in plastic wrapping as fat and acid may absorb chemicals.

- Avoid wrapping food in plastic wrap – use greaseproof paper and paper bags.

- Avoid pesticides by buying organic produce where possible. If you buy non-organic fruit and vegetables, either peel them or soak them in a solution of cider vinegar or sodium bicarbonate to remove some of the residues.

- If you eat meat, poultry and dairy produce, make sure it is organic.

- Don't smoke and avoid smoky atmospheres.

- Get a water filter fitted or use a jug water filter.

- Consider alternatives to the contraceptive pill or HRT.

- Many fish contain high levels of PCBs. Bass and Bluefin tuna are best avoided. Swordfish is high in mercury so is also best avoided. Other fish may contain smaller amounts of toxins. It is advisable to vary the fish you eat and avoid farmed fish and endangered species as much as possible.

- Eat plenty of fibre. Fibre aids in the removal of toxins and old hormones from the body. It is found in whole grains, beans, lentils, fruit and vegetables.

- Use natural skin and body products wherever possible.

- Use natural cleaning agents for doing the dishes, clothes washing and cleaning the house. Chemical nasties to avoid include: ammonia, chlorine, monoethanolamine, glycol ethers, alkylphenol ethoxylates, phthalates, perchlorethylene, sodium hydroxide and triclosan. Good, natural alternatives include: vinegar, lemon juice, tea tree oil, salt, club soda, borax, soapy water, baking soda and good old-fashioned elbow grease!

Feed your ... bump

So you're pregnant? Congratulations! Hopefully you've been following a healthy diet anyway. But there are two (or more) of you to think of now, so your diet needs some extra considerations.

   If your diet is already healthy and nutritious, then that is fantastic. However, it's worth reminding yourself why you need to be extra-aware during pregnancy. For a start, your body requires more protein, so include some with every meal. Good sources include organic white meat, fish (apart from those listed above), well-cooked, free-range eggs, tofu, beans, peas, lentils, quinoa, amaranth and sprouted legumes and seeds. Protein absorption from plant-based foods can be increased by combining them in the same meals. So try combining whole grains with legumes or nuts and seeds (for example lentils with brown rice, make your own haricot healthy baked beans on rye toast, bean burgers with millet risotto, tahini on oat cakes).

You need at least five portions of fresh fruit and vegetables daily – more if you can – as they're so rich in vitamins, minerals and packed with protective antioxidants. When you're cooking vegetables, steaming and water stir-frying are the best methods to preserve nutrients. Drinking freshly pressed vegetable juices will help to increase your vitamin and mineral intake. Fruit juices are best diluted with water as they have a high natural sugar content.

Eating complex carbohydrates will help to sustain your energy levels and maintain blood-sugar balance. They also contain plenty of fibre, which is important for preventing constipation – a problem you may come across during pregnancy (see page 174). Best sources are whole grains such as rye bread, brown rice, millet, pot barley, buckwheat noodles and sugar-free muesli.

If you want the very best brain, eye and vision development for your baby, you need foods rich in essential fatty acids, especially omega-3 fats. Good sources include oily fish (don't exceed two portions a week), pumpkin seeds, walnuts, dark leafy green vegetables and unrefined, cold-pressed seed oils such as flaxseed oil or hemp seed oil.

Your calcium needs increase in pregnancy, so include calcium-rich foods such as live natural yoghurt, dark leafy greens, sea vegetables, tofu, chickpeas, sesame seeds, tahini, almonds and dried figs. If you're eating dairy products, always opt for organic and minimize calcium-containing foods that are high in saturated fat such as whole milk, cream and full-fat cheeses. Vitamin D is needed for proper calcium absorption. Although this vitamin is found only in a small number of foods, the body can produce it naturally from sunlight – so make sure you get outdoors every day. If you are pregnant, your doctor may recommend vitamin D supplements, but do not take them otherwise.

Now you're expecting, your blood volume has increased. Iron is a major component of red blood cells, so you need more of it. Although red meat is high in iron, it can also be high in saturated fat. Healthier, iron-containing choices include beans, lentils, chickpeas, millet, well-cooked, free-range eggs, dark green leafy vegetables, poultry, nettle teas, raisins and prune juice – so there's plenty of choice for vegetarians and vegans. To increase your iron absorption, consume foods or drinks that are rich in vitamin C at the same time.

You probably know that folic acid is vital before and during the first twelve weeks of pregnancy, and as well as taking a supplement (see below), try to include foods high in this B vitamin, such as broccoli, Brussels sprouts, asparagus, peas, brown rice and chickpeas.

Healthy snacks will ward off hunger pangs, keep blood-sugar levels balanced and, believe it or not, help if you have morning sickness, too (see page 189). My top snacks are fresh or stewed fruit, dried (unsulphured) fruit with nuts and seeds, rye bread or oat cakes with nut butter or hummus, live natural yoghurt, vegetable crudités with hummus or olive tapenade.

Finally, drink at least eight glasses of bottled or filtered water daily to help to control food cravings and to maintain hydration levels (drink more if you are moving around a lot or it's a hot day). Remember, you need more fluids now than you normally drink. Good herbal teas during pregnancy include peppermint (for indigestion), chamomile (for insomnia) and nettle (to boost energy and provide iron).

Foods to avoid

Now I'm not one to start with what's forbidden, but in pregnancy I'm afraid this is one thing it's important to get straight from the off. If I don't tell you, your GP or midwife soon will!

There are various foods that you should avoid because they might make you ill or harm your unborn baby. These include:

- Foods that may contain the bacteria listeria, such as unpasteurized cheeses (Camembert, Brie, chèvre and blue cheeses) and meat-based pâtés.

- Foods that may contain salmonella such as raw or partially cooked eggs and undercooked meats. Also foods made using raw eggs such as mayonnaise, salad dressings, some desserts and ice creams.

- Liver products and supplements containing fish liver oils as they can be excessively high in vitamin A, a build-up of which could be harmful during pregnancy.

- Certain types of fish including shark, swordfish and marlin. In addition, have no more than two portions of oily fish (tuna, mackerel, sardines or trout) a week. These fish contain traces of mercury – a toxic metal.

- Raw shellfish as they sometimes contain harmful bacteria and viruses.

- All alcohol and caffeine.

- Peanuts – if the baby's father, brothers or sisters have a nut allergy. Avoid any foods to which there are allergies in the family.

- Foods that are generally unhealthy such as fried foods; foods high in saturated fats; sugar and all foods that contain sugar; refined grains, white rice and white flour products such as white bread and white pasta; junk foods and table salt.

My key supplements for pregnancy

Do not take any supplements or herbs during pregnancy itself without the approval of your GP or health practitioner.

Take folic acid (400mcg) daily from two or three months before you hope to conceive until the twelfth week of pregnancy as this B vitamin helps to prevent neural tube defects such as spina bifida. You can take it through the entire pregnancy. Alternatively, take a good multi-nutrient formula specifically designed for pregnant women as it will contain vital nutrients for this time of life, especially folic acid, calcium, iron and zinc.

Pregnant women do need extra essential fatty acids so supplement with a tablespoon of flax oil daily. Or add linseeds to salads and soups. Two tablespoons daily is perfect.

Probiotics will aid regular bowel function and improve nutrient absorption.

I'd strongly recommend taking a superfood supplement containing wheat-grass juice or powder, or spirulina – it's a useful way of boosting your nutrient intake, especially if you find you go off certain types of food at times.

Feed your . . . newborn

I'm all for good nutrition from day one. It is strongly believed that breastfeeding improves a baby's development and growth, immunity, intelligence, organ strength, helps to prevent allergies and may even promote a calmer disposition. And for you? Breastfeeding can be relaxing, calming, bonding, emotionally nurturing, good for your immunity and for balancing your hormones (reducing your risk of post-natal depression and other problems). But it is draining nutritionally for the mother so you do have to beef up your nutritional support by eating properly and using superfoods to make sure you get enough nourishment.

I must also stress though that it is always a mother's choice when it comes to feeding her baby. Don't beat yourself up if it doesn't come easily to you, or if you prefer not to do it. But do be open to the idea. Even if your mother did not breastfeed you or family members frown on the idea, be true to yourself. If you can do it, then do it.

Because breast milk is designed for human babies, it's much easier for them to digest than formula or cow's milk, and contains at least 100 different compounds not found in formula. It's especially rich in the nutrients required for brain development, healthy bacteria for the baby's digestive system and iron and zinc – both essential nutrients for growth. During the first few days of life, it is particularly important that the baby receives a substance from the milk called colostrum, which contains all the maternal antibodies to help to fight early infections, illness and disease.

It also releases the necessary hormones to instruct your uterus to clamp back down to its pre-pregnant size and burns huge amounts of extra calories – in other words, it's a brilliant, natural weight-loss aid.

If you're going to breastfeed, I highly recommend taking the herb agnus castus. It stimulates production of prolactin, a hormone necessary for milk production. Start roughly one week before you anticipate giving birth and continue for two weeks. Take for three weeks if you feel the quantity of your milk is subsiding.

Boob-boosting tea formula

This special boob-boosting tea formula is a superb way of increasing your milk supply:

You will need some dried leaves of **fennel, marshmallow root, fenugreek, aniseed, coriander and blessed thistle**. The majority of the formula (approx 70 per cent) should be split evenly between the fennel and marshmallow root and then fenugreek should be about 20 per cent, with the other three combining for the remaining 10 per cent of the formula. Pour boiling water over the herbs. Infuse (let sit) for ten minutes and drink.

Alternatively, simmer **1–2 tsp of fenugreek seeds** in $\frac{1}{2}$ pint water for 15 minutes. Drink the tea and eat the seeds.

Important lifestyle advice for the reproductive years

Exercise

Hopefully, you developed good exercise habits in your teens and take part in some form of physical activity at last five days a week. If not, it's certainly not too late to start. The activity needs to be moderate intensity, so you work up a bit of a sweat and feel slightly puffed, and last at least thirty minutes. Don't forget it can be incorporated into your daily life, so if it seems like a tall order, remember brisk walking to and from work or the school run, doing some gardening or vigorous housework or DIY would all count. Most of my clients gradually work up to sixty minutes a day of exercise. It does not have to be all at once.

As well as cardiovascular (aerobic) exercise, which works your heart and lungs, you also need to be incorporating weight-bearing exercise to build and protect your skeleton (you're still building bone mass until you're about thrity-five).

Regular exercise will also keep your weight in check, improve your mood, energy levels and quality of sleep.

Addictive behaviours

A lot of young folk like to experiment, to be part of the crowd and be accepted. Risk-taking behaviour like smoking, drinking alcohol or trying drugs is certainly not unknown in the teens and early twenties. Unfortunately, if you're not careful, it can easily become a habit. And then, if you're under particular psychological stress (as many women in their twenties and thirties are from time to time), a habit can become a dependency or addiction. Older people can develop addictive habits, too, it's not just a concern in your teens and twenties. My advice, of course, is never to let addictive behaviours become a habit. Smoking is vile and foul and is becoming less and less socially acceptable – at last – but the UK still has a big drinking culture and it's easy to kid yourself you're not dependent when you share a bottle of wine a night, or have one or more nights on the town a week. Don't smoke, don't touch drugs and don't even think of exceeding the government recommended limit of 14 units of alcohol a week. Frankly, that 14-unit limit is far too high. Most important of all, be a leader not a follower. Do not drink because the crowd drinks and don't drink to be accepted. Be your own person. Drinking alcohol should be for special celebratory occasions if at all. You don't need it.

The good news is that there's help out there if you do need help kicking a habit – your GP's surgery or phonebook will have details of local services and the NHS has plenty of great advice online. The sooner you do it the better.

Sex and contraception

Sex in your twenties and thirties is about discovering what you like, increasing your confidence and your repertoire. Crucially, it's also about staying safe and, unless baby-making is your aim, protecting yourself from pregnancy.

These days there are so many choices when it comes to contraception. You can use condoms, female condoms, a diaphragm, cervical cap and spermicide. Then there are the hormonal contraceptives – oral contraceptive pills, intra-uterine devices (IUDs) like the Mirena coil, injections, patches and implants. You can opt for natural family planning methods, which involve knowing your cycle and only having sex when you're not likely to be fertile (although as this is obviously less reliable it should only be an option when pregnancy wouldn't be a total catastrophe for you!). And, for those who are sure they never want children, there's sterilization. In women, this involves an operation where the Fallopian tubes are either clipped (which can be reversed) or cut (which cannot be reversed); in men it's the vas deferens, the tube that delivers sperm from the testes to the penis, which is clipped or cut. This needs careful consideration. If you change your mind, reversal is rarely available on the NHS and is not always successful. Sterilization is not something I would recommend and your medical doctor is very unlikely to suggest it to you if you are otherwise healthy.

Each contraceptive method has its advantages and disadvantages and some are more reliable than others. As a rule, hormonal methods are more effective – but they also have more side effects and possible long-term health risks. You need to find the type that's best for you – taking into account your age, health, relationship and how much of a disaster an unwanted pregnancy might be – and that's a very personal decision. It's also a decision you need to review over the years, as your life situation changes.

Most GPs are fully trained in contraception, but there are other sources of information on contraception, like your local family planning clinic where you can speak to medical experts and get all the latest information.

Don't forget that whatever method you choose, you will need to use condoms to protect yourself from sexually transmitted infections (STIs) (see below). Don't have sex without a condom unless you've both had an STI check which means you will need to see STI test results. I know you may think I am being crazy about this but it's your health and life that are at stake. It's that important. If you care enough about yourself you will see it my way, too.

Relaxation and stress relief

A woman can experience stress at any age. Depending on your personal situation and circumstances, whatever decade you are in can be a busy one. Pressure comes from all sides – work, partners, children, friends and family. Many of us thrive on this pressure – after all we're women, we can multi-task! But getting the balance right between your various commitments is important for your physical and emotional health. (See also the section on stress, page 165).

Make sure work commitments don't spill into your private time. Decide when you are going to start and stop work each day and avoid having this stretched. Try to set boundaries and not to bring work home. If that's impossible from time to time, only work in one part of the house – not your lounge and never your bedroom. Weekends and holidays are important for relaxing and refuelling. Spend quality time with your friends, partner and family each week. Set time aside for being with your children, having some intimate moments with your partner and being there for your friends.

But make yourself a promise for life that you'll make time just for you, each day, too. This may be spent exercising, doing yoga, going for a walk, reading, going to an afternoon screening at the pictures. Just make sure your needs are prioritized – even if it's just half an hour soaking in the bath with the door locked!

Finally, spend time outside every day, whatever the weather, preferably somewhere green. And don't forget to breathe – I mean really breathe! Take deep breaths with full inhalations and exhalations. It's instantly relaxing and one of the quickest ways to tell your body and mind that everything is OK. What could be better for the soul than taking five minutes to sit on a park bench, breathe deeply and feel the sun on your face?

Health checks and tests

It's never too early to get into the habit of checking your breasts. In fact it's vital to know what's normal for you at different stages of your menstrual cycle, so you can easily spot and report lumps or other changes. Read more about checking your breasts on page 309.

Cervical smear tests

The NHS Cancer Screening Programme (cancerscreening. nhs.uk) is attended by almost four million women a year and saves 4,500 lives every year. All women aged twenty-five to forty-nine (twenty in Scotland and Wales), are invited for free cervical smear tests every three years (then every five years from fifty to sixty-four). It's essential that you're registered with a GP in order to receive your invitation, so check you are – it's easy to forget if you've moved areas when going away to college or university, say. Make sure, also, that you don't ignore your invitation – phone up and make that appointment right away. (The ideal time is mid cycle, so about two weeks after your last period started.)

There's some dispute over when women should start being screened, so you may like to have a test privately if you're under twenty-five – especially if you've been sexually active from a young age. Some women also choose to have private tests more frequently than every three years.

The test is usually carried out at your GP's surgery by your medical doctor or practice nurse, but you can also be screened at your local family planning clinic or genito-urinary medicine (GUM) clinic. The test uses liquid-based cytology to pick up any changes in cells on the cervix which, if left untreated, may eventually develop into cancer. Not all changes develop into cancer. Cervical cancer is one of the few cancers that is preventable, because screening picks up pre-cancerous changes before they have a chance to become cancer. The smear test can prevent 70 per cent of cervical cancers.

It's thought 99 per cent of cervical cancers are linked to infection with the sexually transmitted human papilloma virus (HPV) – but you should always attend screening, even if you are gay or have not been sexually active with a man for some time.

A test takes just a few minutes – it won't hurt but might be a little uncomfortable if you're tense, so try to relax and breathe deeply. You'll be asked to take off your underwear and lie back on a couch with your knees drawn up and legs apart; not the best position, I know. But no need to feel embarrassed. The medical doctor or nurse will insert an instrument called a speculum into your vagina to keep it open, so they can see the neck of your cervix. They'll collect a sample of cells from your cervix, using a brush. These will be put into a pot of liquid and sent to a lab to be examined.

Your results will be sent to the surgery or clinic where you had your test and you may also receive a letter. Your clinic will contact you if there's any cause for concern, but may not do so if the results were normal. Nine out of ten smears are normal, so you'll simply be recalled for your next routine smear in three or five years' time. Remember, less than one in 1,000 smear test results show an invasive cancer – it's very rare.

Sexual health screening

Some common misconceptions about being tested regularly for STIs: the nurse who does your cervical smear will pick up anything that's amiss; you haven't got any symptoms so you don't need tests; you haven't had many sexual partners; you're married; you always use condoms . . .

I could go on. None of the above constitutes a good reason for never having had a full sexual health screening. If you are sexually active, you need to be screened. A cervical smear is not an STI screening; not all STIs have symptoms (yet they do all have consequences); it doesn't matter how many or how few partners you have, it only takes one infected person to pass on an STI. Even if you're in a long-term, monogamous relationship, you should both get the all clear before you stop using condoms. And even though condoms are a must, be aware that some STIs can also be passed orally or (in the case of HPV or herpes) through genital to genital contact which means areas that aren't necessary covered by the prophylactic. You should also get a clean bill of sexual health before trying for a baby, as some STIs can complicate labour or be passed on to your child.

I know this might sound like a lecture and I'm sorry, but I have to hammer this home. STIs are on the increase and they're not just annoying or embarrassing. They can have serious consequences for your long-term health or fertility. In the case of herpes or HIV, they'll be with you for life. Why risk it?

You can be screened at your GP's surgery, an STI, genito-urinary medicine or Well Woman clinic, or pay to be screened privately. Tests are straightforward blood, urinary, cervical or vaginal swab tests – quick, easy and painless. Treatment, if necessary, is usually straightforward, too, and you'll be advised when to return for re-screening. Find out more on page 155.

Ovulation tests

Ovulation tests can be bought from your chemist and may be useful if you are trying to conceive or are not sure if you're ovulating every month. They don't actually tell you how fertile you are or whether you have any particular hormonal problems (for information on that, see 'Female hormone panel tests', page 122).

You can only become pregnant during a couple of days of your cycle when the mature egg is released from the ovaries (ovulation). However, sperm may survive in a woman's body for up to forty-eight hours after ejaculation. So you should have sex up to forty-eight hours before you ovulate.

The most popular type of ovulation test involves a urine test. About two to three days before ovulation, there is a surge of luteinizing hormone (LH) which can be detected in your urine. This is useful as it can give you a day or two of warning as to when you are most likely to conceive. Saliva tests measure the oestrogen levels in your saliva and may not be as accurate as the urine tests.

Note, though, that neither of these tests can tell you that you've definitely released an egg, or that the egg is healthy.

'Make yourself a promise for life that you'll set aside time just for you.'

Female hormone panel tests

These are generally only available privately, but they may provide a more accurate picture of your hormonal fluctuations over a month than many of the tests available on the NHS. Usually, a full test involves collecting saliva samples over one whole menstrual cycle (this can be done at home) which are then sent to a lab for analysis. This puts the test at an advantage over blood tests which are usually taken in isolation, giving just a snapshot of the hormonal situation and not reflecting fluctuations over the month.

Saliva tests also measure the free, or active, hormones, whereas blood tests measure the total amount of each hormone (which is not indicative of the amount of those hormones that are actually functional).

They don't really add anything helpful in terms of actually getting pregnant but they may be interesting. Many hormone tests are actually available on the NHS, including: oestradiol, FSH, LH, testosterone. The tests can expose hormone imbalances but they won't help you to work out your cycle.

You can discuss with your medical doctor what the results mean in terms of getting pregnant.

Food intolerance tests

It is estimated that 60 per cent of the UK population suffers from unsuspected food reactions, or 'intolerances' that can cause a wide range of health problems. Symptoms can be very wide-ranging and intolerances to different foods can contribute to complaints ranging from arthritis to eczema to migraines.

A food intolerance can weaken your resistance to common ailments and other conditions, making you feel generally unwell without any really obvious cause.

Should I consider a food intolerance test?
There are many reasons for you to investigate food
intolerances or sensitivities. The list below covers the
widespread effects associated with food intolerance.
If you regularly experience any of the following
symptoms, this may be the test for you:

- Abdominal pain
- Aches and pains
- Acne
- Anxiety
- Bloating
- Constipation
- Chronic fatigue
  syndrome
- Depression
- Diarrhoea
- Dizziness
- Eczema
- Fatigue
- Irritable bowel syndrome
- Itching
- Fluid retention

- Headaches
- Hyperactivity
- Loss of appetite
- Migraine
- Nausea
- Rashes
- Respiratory symptoms
- Restless leg syndrome
- Rhinitis
- Sinusitis
- Stomach cramps
- Tension
- Tiredness
- Urticaria
- Weight loss
- Wheezing

What is the difference between allergies and intolerances? Allergies and intolerances are both types of adverse reaction to food.

A food allergy is when the body mistakes the protein in the food as dangerous and produces antibodies to fight it. This causes a reaction to the food. When that food is eaten, the body releases chemicals, for example histamine, which can produce rashes, swelling, asthma, vomiting, hay fever or worse. Allergic reactions can be immediate after contact with an allergen or may appear over a couple of days. The reaction can be slow and minor to severe. You will generally know straight away if you are allergic to something because the swiftness of the reaction allows you to identify the link between cause and effect.

A food intolerance is an adverse reaction to food that does not involve the immune system. An **intolerance** or **sensitivity** may cause reactions that can occur between one and forty-eight hours later. These are much harder to identify – if something you ate at lunchtime causes you to be tired in the afternoon, or a sandwich gives you a headache two days after you ate it because you have a wheat intolerance, you are unlikely to link the two events without careful investigation.

'You have the potential to be in the best physical health!'

What does food intolerance testing involve?
One method is to rely on an elimination-and-challenge
diet and a symptoms history for diagnosis. This would
involve eliminating the possible culprit foods for a certain
period of time – around six weeks is recommended – during
which time you monitor changes in symptoms. After six
weeks you can reintroduce the food and watch for reactions.
Your pulse rate may increase or previous symptoms may
flare up.

Other tests include skin-prick blood tests and kinesiology.
These vary in their accuracy. It is often best to consult with
a nutritional therapist if you want help establishing whether
you have a food intolerance and what the best course of
action may be.

Food intolerance tests usually involve a simple finger-
prick blood test that can be carried out in the comfort of your
own home. Usually a test kit is sent to you in the post, which
contains everything you need to collect your blood sample.
Once you have collected your sample, you simply post it to
the laboratory for analysis.

See www.gillianmckeith.info for food intolerance testing.

For allergy testing see your GP.

Reproductive years – energy synchronization

It'll come as no surprise that I would like you to feel free to focus on your reproductive energy centre at various times during these decades. The main energy centre associated with the reproductive years is the second or sacral chakra, located between your pubic bone and your navel, and it is associated with the colour orange. This is where much of your energy is centred at this time of life.

Creativity, reproduction, intimacy and sexuality are associated with this energy centre. The production of new life is an ultimate creation, but it is not the only way to be creative. Being creative in any way you enjoy can help to shift blockages and free up energy. That's why taking up dance, art, creative writing, sculpting, music or anything else is so beneficial.

Likewise, freeing up energy in this region could possibly make it easier to conceive. But making babies is not the only reason to turn your attention to this chakra. It is essential to synchronize energies in every part of the body for a fulfilled and healthy life.

What's more, it is particularly important that your energy is synchronized in the reproductive region, since this energy centre is a focal area of the body and involved in so many other aspects of life.

Anyone can have blockages in this region, at any time. Our hectic modern lives – overwork, too much responsibility – are to blame. It's easy to forget about ourselves and that's when we're most prone to hindering our natural energy flow.

Here are some tips to help balance energy flow in your reproductive region:

- Drink warm water and lemon juice first thing in the morning. Drink still water and nettle tea throughout the day, but never ice-cold beverages.

- Eating fruit, such as grapefruit, before breakfast has a cleansing effect on the system.

- Apricots, peaches and avocados can be added into smoothies, too.

- All vegetables are good but be sure to include squash, asparagus, Brussels sprouts, pumpkins, sweet potatoes, swedes and carrots. Snack on seeds, including raw shelled hemp, pumpkin, linseeds, chia and sunflower seeds. The grains, quinoa and millet are good – Brazil nuts, too.

- Use vanilla seeds and pods, cinnamon and sweet cicely for seasonings.

- Essential oils to balance this centre are cardamom, mandarin, neroli, orange and sandalwood.

- Be creative. Sing, dance, paint, draw, sculpt, write – anything that takes your fancy. Who cares if you're any good at it – just enjoy it!

- Do any form of regular, moderate exercise that's fun for you: walking, stretching, trampolining, swimming, boxing, t'ai chi chi gung – you choose. Any form of dance is particularly good. Give belly-dancing, hip-hop, jazz, flamenco, ballroom or ballet a go. Most importantly, mix it up and exercise regularly.

- All you need is love! I'm not (necessarily) talking about sexual intercourse or physical sexual impulses. True love is about allowing the free flow of energy on all levels; opening up to who you really are at your core, freeing your spirit. So it's important to choose your friends wisely. If a friend or partner doesn't feel like a real friend, maybe they're not so good for you? If you feel that a friend is perpetually blocking your free flow of energy, you need to take a serious look at the situation and the 'friendship'. Maybe it's time to move on. If your friend or partner allows you to be the real (free-flowing) you, then this opens the flow of love further. True love requires that you love yourself first and foremost – then you're able to share it with others. The energy of love is the most healing element in our existence, and for this reason it is imperative that we free our energy centres so that we can feel and experience the flow of love, unencumbered.

Energy balancing synchronization

The following exercise need not take you more than five minutes to do. But I'd like you to do it each and every day, preferably once in the morning and again in the evening.

1 Lie down in a comfortable position in a quiet room and close your eyes.

2 Listen to your breathing. Let your body do the breathing; you don't need to force it. Your body naturally breathes. You are simply developing your imagination and freeing your energy in the process. Imagine that you can see your breath slowly coming into your whole body, filling your feet and legs, tummy, private area, chest, back, arms, neck, head; and then imagine you see the slow exhale of the breath leaving your body. Watch the inhalations and exhalations for about a minute. You are visualizing and observing your breath.

3 Once relaxed, imagine a ball of orange light slowly swirling around your reproductive region, large enough to include the navel, sometimes referred to as the 'fourth chakra'. Visualize this swirling ball of orange light for about one minute. If you wish, you can imagine an amazing, illuminated orange flower instead of the swirling ball, or feel free to alternate the visualizations. Continue to listen to your breath. I will say to you now that if the colour orange does not come in, do not worry about that at all. White is fine or just simply focus on the breath.

4 Then imagine that this swirling orange ball or flower, originating in your reproductive region, starts to grow and flow throughout your body. Your abdomen, back, legs, feet, arms, neck and head all get filled with the most vibrant orange illumination. It's so bright that it can fill the room, too, if you desire. You need only to use your imagination here. You choose.

Now just 'be' with this beautiful, vibrant light, and be with yourself as you continue to lie down for as long as you choose.

'Be creative. Sing, dance, paint, draw, sculpt, write . . . Who cares if you're any good at it – just enjoy it!'

Reproductive years – common conditions

Bacterial vaginosis

Bacterial vaginosis (BV) is an overgrowth of bacteria in the vagina – usually several different types of bacteria rather than one specific infection. One in ten women has BV at some time in their life, although this is a conservative estimate as it's possible for women to be infected without experiencing any symptoms – it could be as many as one in three.

Symptoms, when they do occur, include vaginal discharge which is usually white or grey in colour and may have a fishy odour. The discharge may be heaviest after sex or just after a period. Unlike thrush, BV does not cause itching.

A healthy vagina contains lots of beneficial bacteria that help protect against harmful infections such as candida. In BV, the balance between healthy and unhealthy bacteria is disrupted and the unhelpful bacteria thrive and flourish. The vagina is naturally acidic and anything that alters this pH can encourage unhelpful bacteria to proliferate. This includes using perfumed toiletries which have an alkaline effect and excessive washing of the vagina, particularly with antibacterial soaps. Semen can also irritate as it's alkaline.

If you have BV during pregnancy, you're at increased risk of complications such as premature birth, miscarriage and infection of the womb after the birth. Complications are also more likely to arise if you have surgery during a BV infection. So although it might seem like a minor irritation, it's important to recognize it, treat it and take steps to prevent a recurrence.

If you suspect BV, your GP will take a vaginal swab to send to the lab for testing. Conventional treatment involves either a single dose or a course of antibiotics. Alternatively, antibiotic or lactic-acid gels can be used inside the vagina to restore balance.

What you can do

Supporting the immune system and the body's bacterial balance through diet and lifestyle can help to clear the infection and prevent recurrences.

Gillian's diet and supplement tips

- Avoid sugar, caffeine, refined foods, saturated fats, alcohol, soft drinks and chocolate. These can all stress the immune system and provide an environment in which unhealthy bacteria can thrive.

- Garlic has anti-bacterial properties so include it in your diet, raw if possible. Likewise the herbs oregano and thyme.

- Eat a fibre-rich diet to encourage the growth of good bacteria. Good sources include oats, brown rice, quinoa, fruit, vegetables and pulses.

- Supplement with probiotics such as acidophilus. This is a beneficial bacterium that should be present in the vagina. Supplementing with it can help to re-establish healthy bacteria and promote health generally. It will also be useful if you've taken antibiotics to clear the BV, as these can often give you thrush (see page 169). Pessaries containing acidophilus can also be used to re-populate the area with good bacteria locally, and you can apply live, natural yoghurt.

General lifestyle tips

- Avoid douching, using soap, shower gels, bath oils or bubble baths and over-washing your genitals.

- Use condoms to prevent semen upsetting the pH of the vagina.

- Choose underwear in natural fibres like cotton and silk. These allow the skin to breathe and prevent moisture building up (bacteria thrive in warm, moist environments).

- Stop using tampons. These are often made from unnatural fibres that can cause irritation in the vagina and upset bacterial balance. Try organic cotton sanitary towels or moon cups instead. If you must use tampons, buy organic, unbleached ones from a health-food store.

Cervical cancer

Cervical cancer affects around 2,800 UK women a year and is the second most common cancer in women under thirty-five. Thanks to the NHS national cervical screening programme, running since 1967, cases and deaths have reduced dramatically. But it's still vital to be aware of this cancer – how to reduce your risk and how to spot the signs.

Your cervix is the ring of muscle at the top of the vagina that forms the entrance to your womb. It is now known that 99 per cent of all cervical cancers are caused by the sexually transmitted human papillomavirus (HPV). This is incredibly common, with about 80 per cent of people in the UK having the infection at some point in their lifetime. There are more than a hundred types of HPV. Some of these are harmless and symptomless, others may cause genital warts and about thirteen types are linked with cervical cancer.

All girls aged twelve to thirteen in the UK are now offered a vaccination against the two most common cancer-causing strains of HPV (see page 54), and this is slowly being rolled out to all those under the age of eighteen. Other women may choose to have it done privately. As well as HPV infection, other risk factors include:

- Being infected with both HPV and herpes or chlamydia
- Smoking
- Taking the contraceptive pill
- Having a compromised immune system (women with AIDs and HIV or those taking immune-suppressive drugs are at greater risk)
- Having lots of sexual partners or having sex with men who have had a lot of sexual partners
- Giving birth to more than three children
- Having your first child before the age of seventeen

Symptoms may include vaginal bleeding between periods or after sex and sometimes pain during sex. You may notice a heavy, watery discharge that's blood-stained and foul-smelling. It's unusual, however, to notice symptoms of cervical cancer unless you haven't been having regular smear tests.

If you do have symptoms, you'll be referred to a gynaecologist who'll examine your cervix and take a tissue sample (biopsy) for analysis – this process is called a colposcopy. You may also need blood tests, X-rays, CT and MRI scans.

If you are diagnosed with cancer, you may require surgery. Discuss with your medical doctor all the treatment options available to you and any implications these may have for your fertility.

What you can do

It's absolutely essential to use condoms, to attend your cervical smear tests when invited and to return for follow-up checks if required. Cervical cancer is associated with smoking so quit if necessary. If you're twenty-six or under, consider having the HPV vaccination privately (you'll still need to attend your smears) (see page 54). For my tips on reducing your risk of and coping with female cancers, see page 360.

Endometriosis

Endometriosis is a chronic condition in which tissues that ought to develop inside the inner layer of the uterus wall end up outside it. This tissue can migrate into the ovaries and Fallopian tubes, the pelvic cavity and the ligaments that surround the womb. It can even move to the bladder, bowel, vagina and lungs. The rogue tissue behaves as it would inside the uterus, following the rhythm of your menstrual cycle. This can mean bleeding from the vagina, bladder or bowel – but blood inside the pelvis or elsewhere is trapped. This irritates the surrounding tissues and causes inflammation and pain. Eventually it can lead to scarring and cysts and adhesions forming. In some women, this can affect fertility. The classic symptom is pain – often severe – in the run-up to and at the start of your period. Other symptoms can include:

- Pain or a dull ache in the pelvis at other times
- Finding intercourse uncomfortable
- Lower back pain
- Pain on passing urine
- Constipation or diarrhoea

But some women experience few if any symptoms.

Endometriosis is generally a problem that occurs during the reproductive years as the female hormones, particularly oestrogen, are responsible for triggering the tissue growth that is at the heart of the condition. It may start soon after puberty and continue until the menopause – most cases are diagnosed in women between the ages of twenty-five and thirty-five. About 10 per cent of women of reproductive age suffer from endometriosis.

We still don't know for sure what causes the condition, but the following may contribute:

- 'Retrograde bleeding' where menstrual blood flows backwards up the Fallopian tubes and into the pelvic cavity
- Genetic predisposition

Endometriosis can take years to be diagnosed, because the symptoms are easy to confuse with other conditions, such as painful periods, irritable bowel syndrome (IBS) or pelvic inflammatory disease (PID). It's also hard to pick up on a scan so is usually only confirmed by a laparoscopy (keyhole surgery via the abdomen) if severe pelvic pain is an issue.

Conventional treatment usually involves drugs that block the hormone cycle, such as the contraceptive pill – although these have to be stopped if you wish to try for a family. Sometimes surgery is required to remove abnormal deposits and reduce symptoms. Although fertility may be compromised, becoming pregnant usually eases symptoms considerably due to the interruption of the hormonal fluctuations that occur during the menstrual cycle. After pregnancy some women find their endometriosis is permanently cured, but for others symptoms recur. The menopause usually brings an end to the condition.

What you can do
Gillian's diet tips

Although there is limited supporting evidence to suggest a direct link between diet and endometriosis, I believe the following may help to ease symptoms in the long term:

- Base your diet around nutrient-dense wholefoods, such as: soya beans, lentils, tofu, beans, legumes, vegetables, seaweeds, seeds, nuts, brown rice, quinoa, oats, millet and fruit.

- Include foods rich in beta-carotene like pumpkins, squash, yams, sweet potatoes, carrots and apricots.

- You need plenty of oily fish such as salmon, mackerel and tuna, plus linseeds, flaxseeds, nuts and raw shelled hemp seeds – all of which contain anti-inflammatory essential fatty acids. These essential fats are also vital for hormonal balance.

- Pick liver-building foods such as artichokes, sauerkraut, cherries, cauliflower, cabbage, Brussels spouts, broccoli, apples. The liver is often implicated in conditions that indicate hormonal imbalances.

- Eat pineapple for its anti-inflammatory bromelain.

- Choose vitamin C-rich berries like blueberries, raspberries, strawberries and gooseberries. Vitamin C has an anti-inflammatory and healing effect.

- Choose zinc-rich foods such as nuts, fish, eggs, wheatgerm and brewer's yeast. Zinc is needed for hormonal balance and healing.

- Choose magnesium-rich foods such as dark green leafy veggies, parsley, prunes, figs, dates, nuts, seeds, apples, alfalfa, wheat germ, seaweeds: dulse and nori, dandelion greens, kelp, almonds, Brazil nuts, lemons, watercress, millet, artichokes, avocados, cashews, celery, oatmeal, black-eyed peas, lentils, Lima beans, brown rice, kale and spinach. Magnesium deficiency is often implicated in female hormone problems. Magnesium has a relaxing effect on the muscles and nerves so can help to reduce pain and tension.

- Vitamin E has hormone-balancing, healing and anti-inflammatory effects. Good sources include olive oil, avocados and sesame oil.

- Heavy bleeding can lead to iron deficiency and anaemia. Drink nettle tea for its iron content. Other sources of iron include red meat (although this can be high in saturated fat), fish, chicken, lentils, figs, prunes, kombu, watercress and rye.

- Add lots of fresh, green herbs to your cooking as well as the gentle anti-inflammatory spices, turmeric and ginger.

- As well as drinking plenty of water, sip dandelion tea to help the liver, and nettle tea to keep your iron levels up. Add Siberian ginseng tea if you're feeling stressed.

- Avoid alcohol.

- Sugary baked goods and sugar will create inflammation in the body.

- Avoid coffee as it may inhibit mineral absorption and disrupt female hormone balance, possibly worsening the symptoms.

Supplement and herb tips

Always consult your medical doctor before taking supplements and check with a herbalist for the correct dosage of herbs.

- If you're not a fan of seaweed, supplement with kelp tablets. Although once you try avocado and cucumber sushi I think you will love it.

- Take flaxseed oil daily for its anti-inflammatory essential oils.

- Agnus castus can help to balance hormones.

- Motherwort helps to ease pain, as may wild yam extract.

- The herb donq quai can help to relieve symptoms by reducing inflammatory compounds.

- Take a vitamin B complex daily to help manage stress.

- Supplement with magnesium in the week leading up to your period to ease cramps.

- Take a probiotic such as acidophilus to get good bacteria into the gut. Keeping your colon healthy will help to deal with excess oestrogen.

General lifestyle tips

- A hot-water bottle or heated pad may help to ease cramps.

- Being overweight has a negative effect on hormonal balance, so you'll suffer more.

- Exercise is essential – it increases circulation, eases cramps, reduces stress, improves mood, stabilizes hormones and keeps your weight down.

Take sitz baths. Easy to do. Fill your bath with only enough hot water to cover your buttocks and hips. Sit in this water for fifteen to twenty minutes tops. Your circulation should improve if you do this regularly. DO NOT DO sitz baths if you have your period or are pregnant.

Do not dry-clean your clothes. Some experts believe women suffering from endometriosis may be sensitive to the solvents used in this process.

Make sure your bowels move daily as congestion in the bowel may exacerbate the symptoms. See section on constipation (page 174) if this is a problem.

Do regular cleanses. Spend one day each month eating mainly fruit and vegetables and drinking warm water, herbal teas and vegetable juices. This helps to reduce congestion, calm inflammation, aid liver function and improve internal cleansing.

Food intolerance

These days, lots of people have food sensitivities. If you go out for dinner with a large group of friends there will usually be someone who doesn't 'do' wheat, or says they're allergic to dairy. Often they're dismissed as fussy or attention-seeking. But I prefer to think that these people are simply taking charge of their own health and choosing to eliminate foods that don't help them feel their best. It's not usually done on a whim, I can assure you.

The fact is, susceptibility to intolerances or allergies – having some sort of adverse reaction to a food – really is increasing. An allergy means you're likely to get an immediate reaction after exposure to the allergen. Common symptoms are hives, rashes, swellings, redness and itching. With food intolerances or sensitivities, you may not notice a reaction for up to forty-eight hours. This makes them much harder to identify as you may not realize your symptoms are related to what you ate. Symptoms are extremely variable and may include digestive problems, fatigue, eczema, headaches, migraines and excess mucus production.

Common food intolerances include wheat and sometimes the other gluten grains such as barley and rye, dairy products, corn and soya. Why might this happen, and why now?

Common theories are:

1   The hygiene hypothesis – children's immune systems are not challenged enough.

2   A decline in breastfeeding.

3   Family history.

There is also some debate over the following:

- Diets lacking in variety mean some foods are eaten every day, sometimes several times a day. Commonly these are wheat and dairy products which may feature as cereal with milk for breakfast, a cheese sandwich for lunch and a pizza or pasta and sauce in the evening. Ironically, this over-reliance might produce an intolerance.

- Overuse of antibiotics may disrupt the gut bacterial balance and compromise digestive function.

- Modern varieties of wheat that are cultivated to be fast-growing and high in gluten may be particularly irritating to the gut for some people.

- Food-processing techniques for bread, for example, do not allow time for the gluten in the flour to be broken down during fermentation in the way that traditional methods would have done.

- Animals are fed grains rather than being largely grass-fed so their milk is of a different composition from that produced a hundred years ago, and many people can't tolerate it.

What you can do

If you wish to avoid a food intolerance, the following dietary advice may help:

Eat a wide variety of foods, making sure you vary your grain intake in particular. Rather than relying on wheat for every meal, try oats, millet, rye, quinoa, buckwheat, corn, brown rice and red rice as alternatives. Spelt and kamut are ancient varieties of wheat that tend to be less allergenic and can be used in a similar way to wheat in many recipes.

Food rotation is worth bearing in mind. This involves leaving four days between eating foods to which you may be sensitive. So, you may include wheat on Monday, oats on Tuesday, millet on Wednesday, quinoa on Thursday, brown rice on Friday and back to wheat on Saturday. If you notice symptoms occurring after you eat a food or on the same day and possibly even into the next day, note down how you feel. There might just be a connection.

Reacting to a food can also be a sign that you are run down. So do make sure that you are eating properly and getting enough sleep. Burning the candle at both ends is weakening to the immune system and can make your body more reactive to all kinds of things.

> Instead of *always* using cow's milk products, try those made from goat's milk, sheep's milk, soya milk, almond milk, rice milk, almond milk and oat milk. These are all available from health-food stores and, increasingly, supermarkets.

> Avoid processed and junk foods. These tend to rely on refined foods and often contain wheat, soya and dairy products.

> Enjoy your food, chew thoroughly and relax when eating. Eating food when you are under stress and not chewing properly puts a strain on the digestive system and may increase your susceptibility to intolerances.

If you're having unexplained symptoms or you think you may be intolerant or allergic to certain foods, there are various tests available. Or you can try a simple elimination diet (if you're not sure what the culprit might be, a nutritionist can help you to devise a balanced elimination diet to try). If you suspect a food intolerance, you need to exclude the offending item for six weeks and then reintroduce it. Keep a detailed food diary and monitor any symptoms.

The supplement L-glutamine may help to minimize reactions to certain foods so try taking it before meals. There is no medical evidence to support this theory but in my own practice, I have found this supplement to be very helpful especially when there are symptoms of leaky gut. L-glutamine can help to heal a damaged gut wall, which may be at the root of some food intolerances.

Building up your immune system is essential. At the same time as any elimination diet, it's worth going on a six-month course of the immune-strengthening herb astragalus. (It is always advisable to consult a medical doctor before embarking on a course of supplements.)

Irritable bowel syndrome

Irritable bowel syndrome (IBS) is a 'functional bowel disorder', meaning that although the intestine looks normal when examined by X-ray or surgery, its behaviour is anything but. Symptoms are unpleasant and varied but usually a combination of tummy pain, gas, bloating, cramping, constipation and diarrhoea. A tell-tale sign is also mucus in your stools. Of course, many of us experience these symptoms from time to time – perhaps as a result of a stomach bug or poor eating. But in IBS the symptoms will be a more regular and upsetting feature of your life. They may be present all the time or come and go, depending on what triggers them.

Sufferers tend to have tummy pain related to bowel habit, i.e. the pain gets worse or better when you open your bowels. A GP's diagnosis usually involves ruling out other possible causes of the symptoms such as Crohn's disease, colitis, diverticulitis and coeliac disease.

What's happening in IBS is that the muscular contractions of the intestinal tract are irregular and the bowels may go into spasm. They may be unnaturally strong or frequent, the nerves in your intestine may be extra sensitive or there may be a change in the way your brain controls these functions. The result is that movement of food and waste through the gut is badly affected. Sufferers can end up malnourished as this condition interferes with the absorption of nutrients. IBS is an extremely common digestive disorder. It tends to afflict young adults, and women are about three times more likely to suffer IBS than men. Many women experience changes in bowel habits during each menstrual cycle. It may be that the changing levels of oestrogen and progesterone affect intestinal function. A lot of female IBS sufferers find their symptoms are worse during menstruation with increased gas, bloating and diarrhoea. Women are also more likely to suffer from anxiety and depression than men, both of which can be triggers for IBS symptoms (likewise eating disorders). There are no known triggers but IBS is linked to the following:

- Food sensitivities
- Poor diet
- Stress
- Eating under pressure or in a rush
- Excessive use of laxatives, antacids or antibiotics
- Carbonated drinks, spicy foods, wheat bran, alcohol and caffeine

What you can do

Sometimes IBS can be mistaken for a more serious condition such as coeliac disease, ulcerative colitis, diverticulitis or Crohn's disease, so do get checked out by your GP.

Conventional treatment for IBS usually involves drugs such as antispasmodics, laxatives, anti-diarrhoeals and even antidepressants. But these don't deal with the cause of the IBS or seek to identify triggers. This condition is one to which I strongly believe a natural approach is the most effective in the long run. You need to find your irritants and deal with them, then nourish your system with good digestive habits, plenty of gut-friendly foods and a stress-free lifestyle (as far as modern life permits).

It's well worth keeping a food and symptom diary for several weeks or even months, to try to identify any foods or drinks that may be triggers. Include emotions and what's going on in your life, too, so you can see if stress is playing a part. There is no one treatment that works for all sufferers of IBS. Causes are usually multi-factorial and the combination of factors that trigger the symptoms may be different for each person with the condition.

Gillian's diet tips

> Practise 'mindful eating' – take time for meals, sit down, turn off the TV and eat slowly. Chew each mouthful really well, only swallowing once it has become liquid. Put your cutlery down between bites. It's not a race.

> Take some deep inhalations and exhalations before you eat to give the body a message of relaxation.

> Make fresh vegetable juices your friends – they're an easy way to boost your nutrient intake, which is likely to be depleted.

> Whole grains, vegetables, legumes and sprouted seeds provide fibre and pass smoothly through the intestinal tract. But go easy on broccoli, cauliflower, onions and cabbage as they may aggravate symptoms.

> Have your whole grains well cooked so that they are soft and gentle on the intestinal tract.

> Snack on dried figs that have been soaked in water to ease constipation.

> Sprinkle linseeds over salads – this will also help to keep you regular and cleanse the bowel.

> Wheat and dairy products are the most common gut irritants, so it's worth eliminating them to see if your symptoms improve. Try almond, hemp, oat or rice milks instead of cow's milk. Replace wheat with rye, oats, millet, quinoa and buckwheat.

> Likewise cut out corn, processed foods, sugars, sweeteners, margarine and red meat for two months and monitor the results. Do not replace sugars with artificial sweeteners as these may have negative effects on many aspects of health.

Other common irritants to beware of include spicy foods, yeast, tomatoes, citrus fruit and citrus juices.

Hot spices such as black pepper and chilli pepper may exacerbate the symptoms but the milder spices and herbs can improve digestion and gut function. Ginger, coriander, cumin, cinnamon, fennel, mint, cardamom and caraway can all help to stimulate the production of digestive enzymes thus aiding the digestive process and movement through the gut.

It's vital to stay well hydrated so drink at least two litres of filtered or mineral water a day, preferably between meals.

Alcohol and caffeine worsen symptoms so should be avoided. Smoking can also interfere with gut function and lead to spasm in the colon.

Drink herbal teas instead (between meals) to help soothe the gut. Camomile, peppermint, slippery elm, lemon balm and fennel teas are good digestive aids. Pau d'arco tea has anti-inflammatory properties and keeps yeasts at bay.

Avoid artificial sweeteners as these can be irritating to the gut.

Supplement and herb tips

Always consult your medical doctor before embarking on a course of supplements and check with a herbalist for the correct dosage of herbs.

Make sure you're getting enough magnesium which can act as a gut relaxant.

Take a vitamin B complex to help you break down your foods.

Supplement with probiotics to help re-establish good bacterial balance in the intestines.

- Drink aloe vera juice before meals to calm inflammation in the gut.

- Two peppermint-oil capsules in between meals may be enough to reduce gas and intestinal spasms.

- I've seen excellent results with gentiana root. Gentiana is a bitter herb which helps to stimulate digestion. You may want to disguise its unpleasant taste in some apple purée or mashed banana.

- Take L-glutamine powder or capsules. Glutamine is used up in large amounts with those who have IBS. One of its jobs is to carry ammonia to the kidneys for excretion. It is also the main fuel of the intestinal cells and is needed to repair and replace the cells of the intestinal wall.

- Triphala tablets can help the gut to function more smoothly, especially if constipation is a problem.

- Milk-thistle tincture supports the liver and elimination processes. Liver function is often implicated in disorders of the digestive tract

- Rice bran oil is very helpful for healing the gut.

General lifestyle tips

- Learn to manage stress and engage in daily relaxation; yoga, t'ai chi, meditation and breathing exercises are all beneficial.

- Massage your abdomen in a clockwise direction, using a few drops of peppermint essential oil combined with an almond carrier oil.

- Some studies have shown hypnotherapy can be helpful for IBS.

Pelvic inflammatory disease

Pelvic inflammatory disease (PID) is an inflammation of the female reproductive organs, including the womb (uterus), Fallopian tubes and ovaries. The most likely cause is a bacterial infection that starts in the vagina and cervix and spreads to the upper reproductive tract. This is usually a sexually transmitted infection (STI), most commonly chlamydia or gonorrhoea. However, it can be caused by an overgrowth of the bacteria that usually reside in the vagina. Other risk factors include a termination of pregnancy, any uterine surgery such as a dilation and curettage (D and C), childbirth or the insertion of an old-style copper intrauterine device (IUD) or 'coil'.

It's possible to have PID for weeks or months without any discernible symptoms, and the speed at which they develop once they start varies from days to weeks. You may experience:

- Pain in the lower abdomen which can range from mild to severe
- Pain during sex
- Heavier, more painful periods
- Bleeding between periods or after sex
- Abnormal vaginal discharge
- Lower back pain
- Fever
- Water retention
- Fatigue
- Feeling generally unwell

PID is serious because, left untreated, it can lead to inflammation, narrowing and scarring of the Fallopian tubes. This makes ectopic pregnancy and fertility problems more likely. The risk of miscarriage, premature birth or stillbirth is also higher in women with untreated PID. In extreme cases, the infection can cause abscesses, pelvic adhesions and Reiter's syndrome, which involves arthritis and inflammation around the eyes.

In some women, pelvic pain can persist after the condition has been treated and they may be prone to reinfection.

The sooner you identify and report symptoms of PID, the sooner you can be treated and the greater the chance your fertility will be unaffected. Your medical doctor should use a combination of vaginal and cervical swabs, internal and external examination to diagnose you. Treatment is usually a week's course of antibiotics. It is important to tell your GP if you might be pregnant as this can affect the choice of antibiotics. You may also be given painkillers. If your symptoms are sudden and severe, you may need to be admitted to hospital for intravenous antibiotics but this is rare. Take a probiotic supplement if you are placed on a course of antibiotics to replenish the good bacteria.

What you can do

To prevent PID, always practise safe sex and use a condom. Follow my dietary and lifestyle recommendations in the STIs overview section (page 155). If you've been diagnosed with PID:

Do not have sex until after the treatment has finished and any pain has subsided.

Make sure any sexual partners you've had in the past six months are tested and treated for infection.

Hot and cold showers can help to boost circulation and decongest the area. Have a warm shower as usual. Then turn the water to cold and use the shower attachment to run the water up your body, starting with your feet. Direct cold water at your pelvic area for 30 seconds. Then switch to warm for a couple of minutes. Alternate back to cold. Do this two to three times, finishing on cold.

- Exercise also improves circulation to the area – a good flow of blood, nutrients and oxygen can aid healing. Walking, swimming and yoga are all suitable exercises. Just avoid exercise if you're in severe pain or having an acute attack of symptoms.

- Specific physical exercises that can help to get energy flowing in this area include pelvic thrusts and circling the hips.

- Castor-oil packs may help to reduce pain and internal inflammation. Saturate a soft cotton cloth with castor oil and apply directly to your lower abdomen. Cover the area with another thick cloth and hold a hot-water bottle on top for an hour or more. Use the packs on three consecutive days each week for three weeks, then have a break for a week.

- For those prone to repeated bouts of infection, put yourself on a six-month course of the herb astragalus (check with a doctor first). This herb is helpful for strengthening immunity.

Polycystic ovarian syndrome

Up to 33 per cent of women in the UK have polycystic ovaries. Of these, about 33 per cent have polycystic ovarian syndrome (PCOS) which is polycystic ovaries plus other symptoms. It is not the cysts themselves that are the problem in PCOS but the symptoms that result from the hormonal imbalances. These include:

- Irregular or light periods or no periods at all
- Fertility problems, due to lack of ovulation
- Weight gain, especially around the middle
- Excessive hair growth (hirsutism), especially on the face, abdomen, legs and chest
- Thinning hair on the head (similar to male-pattern baldness)
- Greasy skin and acne
- Raised LH/testosterone

Having PCOS puts you at increased risk of insulin resistance, type 2 diabetes and gestational diabetes, as well as high blood pressure, high cholesterol and endometrial cancer in later life.

We don't know exactly what causes it, but a number of factors are thought to play a part, including a genetic predisposition and being overweight.

If PCOS is a possibility, your GP should run blood tests to check your hormone levels, and refer you for an ultrasound scan to look at your ovaries.

What you can do

Conventional treatment options will depend on your symptoms and whether or not you're trying for a family. If not, medical doctors often favour the contraceptive pill to regulate periods, suppress cysts, improve skin and reduce facial hair. If you want to have a baby, they may prescribe drugs like clomiphene to kick-start ovulation. You may also be offered drugs to lower your glucose levels to prevent insulin resistance.

It'll come as no surprise that I favour a more natural approach, and believe the symptoms of PCOS respond very well to diet and lifestyle changes.

All doctors will agree, however, that weight loss should be the main lifestyle change.

Gillian's diet tips

Avoid sugar in all its forms. It can 'hide' in many foods under different names. So check the ingredients on all foods you buy and avoid sucrose, dextrose, glucose, maltose, lactose, honey, molasses, malt extract, corn syrup, golden syrup, maple syrup, treacle and high fructose corn syrup. These all trigger the release of insulin. Also avoid artificial sweeteners as these may disrupt appetite regulation.

Swap refined carbohydrates, such as sugary breakfast cereals, white bread, baguettes, white pasta, white rice, crisps and pastries for whole grains such as oats, rye bread and quinoa.

Eat smaller, more frequent meals so that blood-sugar levels remain stable.

Eat protein with every meal or snack. Protein slows the breakdown of carbohydrates into glucose. Combine animal protein with vegetables and salads. Combine plant proteins (nuts, seeds, lentils, beans, soya) with grains and vegetables.

Have fibre with every meal, too – fibre is an indigestible carbohydrate that does not raise blood sugar or insulin. Fibre slows the breakdown of digestible carbohydrates into glucose. Find it in lentils, beans, whole grains, vegetables and flaxseeds.

Fresh, raw or lightly cooked vegetables provide antioxidants, fibre and nutrients needed for health as well as being low in calories and fat. The more you cook a vegetable the faster the carbohydrates it contains will break down into glucose. Also, who likes the taste of soggy vegetables anyway?

Essential fats improve hormone balance. Good sources include oily fish, flaxseed oil, hemp seeds, pumpkin seeds and avocados.

Low-sugar fruits such as apples, blackberries, blueberries, raspberries, cherries and grapefruit are good choices.

Avoid alcohol, caffeine and nicotine – all stimulants that interfere with blood sugar.

Supplement and herb tips

If you're having fertility treatment or are taking hormone-balancing or blood-sugar-balancing medications (such as the pill, hormone-replacement therapy (HRT) or any medication for diabetes or metabolic syndrome), you should consult your medical doctor before following my supplement programme. Check with a herbalist for the correct dosage of herbs.

The mineral chromium is involved in controlling blood-sugar levels and insulin, so a supplement may help to balance them. Suggested dose: one daily.

B vitamins work with chromium to help control blood sugar and produce energy from food. Suggested dose: B complex 50mg daily.

Magnesium may also improve blood-sugar control and energy production. Take only for a short time.

Zinc is needed for good hormone function and the action of insulin.

The herb garcinia cambogia contains hydroxy citric acid (HCA) which may help carbohydrates to be used for energy rather than being converted to fat. It may also help to curb the appetite and reduce weight gain.

Agnus castus is generally hormone balancing and is believed to help to control the release of LH.

- Some herbalists recommend the herb saw palmetto which may act on hormone levels to help to normalize testosterone production – this may be helpful if your symptoms include excess body hair or thinning hair.

- Milk thistle supports good liver function – your liver is vital for the metabolism and breakdown of hormones. It won't rid you of this condition but it may be a helpful adjunct to your healthy diet.

General lifestyle tips

- Maintain a healthy weight – this often helps to reduce high insulin and testosterone levels as well as reducing your risk of developing diabetes and high blood pressure.

- Take daily exercise – exercise improves the cells' response to insulin, helps to normalize appetite and, of course, burns off glucose and fat.

- Get sufficient sleep – seven to eight hours a night is a good target but whatever makes you feel properly refreshed. People who sleep for less than six hours a night are more likely to become resistant to insulin. Aim to get into bed by ten o'clock every night. Going to bed early gives your body the chance to detoxify naturally and you will feel so much better. Try it.

Sexually transmitted infections

Sexually transmitted infections (STIs) are spread through sexual activity. They include:

CHLAMYDIA The fastest spreading STI in the UK. It is caused by the micro-organism chlamydial trachomatis which is transmitted between partners during unprotected sex. It is a potentially serious condition that can affect both men and women. If the disease is not treated it can lead to the development of PID, damaged Fallopian tubes, ectopic pregnancy and infertility. Women infected with chlamydia can infect their babies when giving birth. In the majority of cases, there are no visible symptoms which is why safe sex and regular screening are essential. When symptoms do occur they appear anywhere between seven and twenty-one days after infection and may include: burning or stinging when urinating, vaginal discharge, pain during intercourse and irregular bleeding.

GENITAL HERPES A viral condition caused by the herpes simplex virus. It is highly contagious and can be spread through physical and sexual contact. Areas affected include the skin and mucous membranes of the genitals and rectum and sometimes the mouth. It can also be spread to a baby during childbirth if the mother is infected at the time of labour. Symptoms usually appear about a week after infection but sometimes take longer. Initially, there may be tingling, pain or burning in the infected area. The skin becomes red and blisters appear. The blisters may burst leaving shallow ulcers which may scab and heal over a week or so. Sufferers may also experience swelling of the lymph nodes in the groin, vaginal discharge, painful urination and fever. There is no cure for the herpes simplex virus – once infected you remain a carrier for life.

GENITAL WARTS Caused by the human papillomavirus (HPV) which is highly contagious. They are the most common STI in the UK. Warts may not develop for up to nine months from the time of infection. The virus can be contracted during sex or skin on skin contact and is contagious even if the warts are not visible. Over 50 per cent of women who have sex will be infected with the virus at some point in their lifetime. Symptoms include raised or flat wart-like growths that may occur singly or in clusters. They're found around the vaginal opening, cervix and anus. Lesions may also appear in the mouth or throat. Warts are usually painless but can become itchy or inflamed. It is possible to be infected without any noticeable symptoms.

Symptoms can worsen during pregnancy, if the person has diabetes or if the immune system is compromised. Very rarely, an infected woman can pass the virus on to her baby during childbirth. Although the HPV virus is known to cause cervical cancer (see page 54), these strains are not the same as those that cause warts. Different strains of the virus cause different reactions.

GONORRHOEA Caused by the bacterium *Neisseria gonorrhoeae*, which thrives in warm, moist areas such as the cervix, urethra, mouth and rectum. Gonorrhoea can be passed from a woman to her baby during childbirth. Symptoms usually appear between two to ten days after infection although some people (particularly women) may be infected for months before developing symptoms. If they appear, symptoms may include burning on urination, pus-like, yellowish or bloody vaginal discharge, pelvic or abdominal pain, itching and painful bowel movements.

Nausea, vomiting, fever and chills may occur if bacteria travel through the bloodstream but this is very rare. If left untreated, gonorrhoea can spread to the uterus and Fallopian tubes, which can lead to the development of PID and infertility. If the bacteria travel through the bloodstream, complications such as arthritis may also arise.

HUMAN IMMUNODEFICIENCY VIRUS (HIV) Transmitted via blood, semen and vaginal fluids. The virus attacks your immune system, destroying certain white blood cells called CD4 cells and weakening your resistance to illness. First symptoms of HIV infection usually appear within six weeks and can include: tiredness, aches and pains, fever and a rash. If it is left untreated, you may develop weight loss, swollen glands, herpes and yeast infections, diarrhoea and night sweats. If the virus manages to reduce the number of CD4 cells to the point where your immune system starts to fail, you can develop acquired immunodeficiency syndrome (AIDS). The body may be unable to resist infections and cancers such as tuberculosis, pneumonia and lymphoma.

SYPHILIS This used to be called 'the pox'. In the past it was a very common disease that could sometimes be fatal. Unfortunately, in the past few years the number of people contracting the condition is rapidly increasing again.

Caused by the bacterium *Treponema pallidum*, it's contracted through close bodily contact or sexual activity. It spreads through the sores of the infected person into the skin of the other person. The sores are not always visible as they can be internal.

It usually takes between two to six weeks after infection before symptoms appear. Primary symptoms include small infectious sores, called chancre, that appear at the points where the bacteria entered the body. This is usually around the genital area. Up to six months after initial infection the sores tend to disappear and a non-itchy rash appears. This is the most infectious stage. The rash may have small brown sores and it can spread all over the body. Other symptoms may include hair loss, headaches, fever, sore throat and swollen glands.

Wart-like growths may also develop around the genitals. These symptoms may come and go for a year or so and may disappear without treatment.

If untreated syphilis can last for years and damage the heart, brain, joints, bones, eyes and nervous system. Blindness, paralysis, mental health problems, heart disease and death are all possible outcomes. Syphilis can be passed from a mother to her unborn baby.

What you can do

The same piece of advice is key for all STIs – prevention is better than cure. Use a condom when having sex, even if you are taking other contraceptives such as the pill. This is imperative. Used correctly, both the male and female condom can usually offer protection from most STIs. The only exception is if you're in a long-term, monogamous relationship and you've both been tested and given the all-clear for all STIs.

It's important that you go for testing in between sexual partners, too – and make sure any new partners have been screened and that you see the test results. I am serious here. Never, and I mean *never*, play Russian roulette with your body and your sexual health. If a partner refuses to get tested, dump that partner! They are obviously not being honest with you or hiding something. Do not take the risk. It is your life I am talking about here.

If you are found to have an STI, you must follow your GP's advice and have the recommended treatment, which may involve topical or oral antibiotics or other preparations, minor surgery or longer-term care, as well as future precautions.

It's essential that you avoid having penetrative sex until you have been retested and are clear of the infection. Your partner should also be tested and treated and you should inform any previous partners who may have been infected.

Here is my generic diet and lifestyle advice for anyone with any sort of STI:

Gillian's diet tips

- Support your immune system with lots of fresh fruit and vegetables. Eat at least eight portions of fruit and vegetables daily to help the body to fight the infection.

- Drink three cups of pau d'arco tea daily to support the immune system and fight the infection.

- Include raw garlic in your diet. Garlic has potent anti-bacterial and anti-viral properties that can help to rid the body of infections.

- Avoid saturated fat, sugar, refined foods, alcohol and caffeine. These may suppress immunity and deplete the body of nutrients.

- Include fibre from whole grains such as brown rice, millet, quinoa, oats, buckwheat and rye. Fibre is needed for cleansing the body and eliminating toxins.

- Include herbs and spices in your meals. In particular oregano and thyme have antibacterial properties and turmeric is a useful anti-inflammatory and antioxidant.

Drink dandelion root coffee to support liver and bowel function. It is important that the organs of elimination and detoxification are working well in order to rid the body of infection.

Supplement and herb tips

Always consult your medical doctor before taking a course of supplements and check with a herbalist for the correct dosage of herbs.

Vitamin C may help to reduce cellular damage caused by some bacteria and viruses. It can be used alongside antibiotics.

Zinc is needed by the immune system and for healing and repair of the body.

Probiotics such as Lactobacillus acidophilus may help to restore healthy bacterial balance after a course of antibiotics.

Immune supportive herbs such as echinacea, astragalus, propolis, goldenseal and barberry can all be taken as tinctures or capsules to aid your body's own defences.

'Going to bed early gives your body the chance to detoxify naturally. Try it.'

Skin cancer

Skin cancer develops when skin cells grow and divide in an abnormal or uncontrolled way. There are various different types of skin cancer depending on which cells are affected.

Non-melanoma skin cancer makes up the majority of skin cancers that are diagnosed. This includes basal cell carcinoma and squamous cell carcinoma. Both can usually be easily treated, rarely spread and are rarely fatal. Treatment may just leave you with some scarring.

The most serious form of skin cancer is malignant melanoma. Left untreated, this can spread quickly around the body and be fatal. There are over 8,000 new cases in the UK each year and the number is rising at an alarming rate. More women are affected than men, perhaps because we tend to be keener on sunning ourselves. 'Lying and frying' in short, sharp bursts – such as on sun beds or on yearly beach holidays – is thought to be the cause of most melanomas.

Melanoma is caused by an overgrowth of the melanocytes in the top layers of the skin. Melanocytes are cells that make melanin when your skin is exposed to the sun. The more melanin produced, the more your skin will darken. Melanoma usually starts as a mole that changes colour, size or shape (or appears to be a new mole). It may become lumpy and ooze or bleed.

There are certain known risk factors that may make you more susceptible to developing skin cancer. These are:

- Exposure to intense ultraviolet light such as sunlight or sun beds
- Excessive or year-round sun exposure
- Having fair skin and an inability to tan
- Having red hair
- Having blue or green eyes

- Having freckly skin or lots of moles
- A family history of skin cancer
- Getting badly sunburnt in the past
- Ageing
- Smoking
- Scarred skin from burns or ulcers
- Radiotherapy
- Compromised immune system

If you have a suspicious-looking mark on your skin, your medical doctor should refer you for investigation. You're likely to need a biopsy – a piece (or all) of the affected skin is removed and tested to see if it is growing and, if so, how fast.

You may also need:

- A sentinel node biopsy, in which the medical doctor removes the nearest lymph node to the melanoma to see if cancer is present there

- X-rays or scans

If it is cancer, treatment will vary according to what type and if it has spread. It may involve:

- Freezing or creams, in the case of small, early skin cancers

- Excision surgery to remove the cancer and some cells around the growth. This is essential treatment for melanoma

- Removal of the nearest lymph nodes if the cancer has spread into them

- Radiotherapy may be used instead of or as well as surgery

- Chemotherapy if the cancer has spread to other body parts

- Immunotherapy if recurrence seems likely

What you can do

Check your skin and moles regularly – ask your partner, friend or relative to check hard-to-see areas like your back. See your GP immediately to check any mole or spot that:

- Increases in size – particularly if it is over 7mm or ¼ in across
- Changes shape, has an irregular edge or is asymmetrical
- Changes colour, gets darker or darkens in patches
- Is itchy or bleeds
- Becomes sore or develops a crust
- Becomes red, swollen or inflamed

Prevention is always better than cure so make sure you:

- Never, ever use sun beds
- Never let yourself burn
- Although some sun is good for you (it's how your body makes vitamin D), you don't need to bake. If you're somewhere hot or the weather forecast tells you the UV risk index is going to be moderate to high, wear UV protective sunglasses and UV skin protection of at least SPF15, stay out of the sun between ten o'clock in the morning and four o'clock in the afternoon and wear a hat to cover up, too

Gillian's diet tips

Foods containing essential fats may be protective. Sources of these include oily fish, hemp seeds, flaxseeds, pumpkin seeds, sunflower seeds, walnuts, avocados and cold-pressed oils such as flaxseed oil.

Turmeric contains curcumin which may protect against skin cancer. It is best processed by the body if taken with fats, so combine it with cold-pressed olive oil or flaxseed oil.

- Drink at least eight glasses of mineral or filtered water daily for overall health.

- Avoid foods that contain toxic trans fats, such as some margarines and many biscuits, cakes and crisps as they are associated with an increase in free radical damage.

- Excess alcohol may be associated with an increased risk.

Supplement and herb tips

Always consult your medical doctor before taking supplements and check with a herbalist for the correct dosage of herbs.

- Resveratrol found in red grapes and cranberries has been found to have anti-skin cancer activity.

- Curcumin found in turmeric and curry powder may help to block the development of melanoma.

- Antioxidants such as selenium and vitamins C and E may all neutralize free radicals that may be produced during exposure to UV light.

- Echinacea and astragalus may help to support the immune system.

General lifestyle tips

- Don't smoke – smoking is associated with an increased risk of many cancers. It depletes the body of nutrients and challenges the immune system. It'll also make you look older!

- Avoid living or working in polluted areas. Pollution increases the risk of developing many cancers, including skin cancer.

Stress

While stress can obviously occur at any point in your life, it's something that often rears its ugly head in your twenties and thirties, as you struggle to balance work, friends, relationships, home life and possibly a family. You could argue that women are exposed to more stress in life as we tend to have more roles to play. The sooner you can adopt a lifestyle and tools to help prevent and deal with stress, the better.

Stress is basically the manifestation of how you respond to difficulties (stressors) in your daily life. Some people are better at dealing with stressors than others as they are less reactive.

Poor response to stress causes a damaging, excessive secretion of the hormones adrenalin and cortisol. These hormones, produced by the adrenal glands, are the 'fight or flight' chemicals – designed to help your body respond to emergency situations. They cause your heart rate to increase, blood-sugar levels to elevate, blood vessels to constrict in some areas, such as the skin, and dilate in others, such as the muscles, and breathing to get heavy. All of this is fine if it is only temporary and the situation warrants such a physical response.

The problem is that your body can misinterpret everyday situations like work problems, a baby crying, relationship issues, financial worries – even traffic jams! – as emergencies. So the stress hormones are released constantly and stay in your system. Stress is a completely natural reaction and our bodies are well designed to deal with it. However, ongoing stress can place a strain on our system. Some studies have shown that this can weaken our ability to fight infection and can leave us more susceptible to illness. Experts estimate that up to 90 per cent of illnesses are stress-related.

Weight problems, mouth ulcers, blood-pressure problems,

stomach ulcers, gastrointestinal disorders, muscle weakness, clogged arteries, impaired memory, depression, anxiety, colds, flus, skin disorders, even repetitive strain injuries have all been connected with high levels of stress hormones over a prolonged period.

What you can do

It's important to try and deal with the source of your stress – whether it is talking to your employer, your family, getting to grips with money issues, or perhaps seeking counselling. But don't underestimate the role of good nutrition and healthy living in helping your body and mind to be less reactive and cope better with whatever life throws at you.

Gillian's diet tips

Brown rice, legumes, parsley and green vegetables are all good sources of B vitamins – vital for good functioning of the nervous system. Think of them as the mood-boosting vitamins. B vitamins play an important role in the health of the adrenal glands.

Sprouts, green vegetables and unrefined cereals and nuts such as almonds contain magnesium which is important for supporting adrenal function and metabolising essential fatty acids. Low levels of magnesium can be associated with nervous tension, anxiety, irritability and insomnia.

Eat asparagus for its antioxidant glutathione and beneficial effect on the liver. Helping the liver may have a positive effect on your mood and stress levels. In traditional Chinese medicine, the liver is seen as the seat of anger. If you feel you have a lot of emotions associated with anger or irritability, either expressed or suppressed, then it is thought to be beneficial to nourish the liver. Avoiding foods and drinks that challenge the liver is a good place to start so cut out alcohol, fatty meats, processed foods and sugar.

Blackberries, strawberries and raspberries are rich in manganese and vitamin C. Insufficient vitamin C can weaken your immune system and make you feel generally stressed and run down.

Herbal teas can help to relieve many stress symptoms by nourishing the central nervous and glandular systems. Find which of the following work best for you: lemon balm, hops, oatstraw, kava, ginseng, chamomile, passionflower, skullcap, liquorice, valerian. Drink cucumber juice, too, for its relaxing effect.

Caffeine has a stimulant effect that can raise blood pressure and increase anxiety.

There may be a link between caffeine intake and high blood pressure and high cholesterol levels. Tea, coffee and colas all act as diuretics, so they flush out many vital nutrients and trace elements.

You may reach for a glass of wine at the end of a hard day but do not use alcohol to deal with stress. Excess alcohol may increase the fat deposits in the heart and decrease the immune function. It also challenges the liver.

Sugar has no essential nutrients. It provides a short-term boost of energy through the body, but the inevitable blood-sugar low that follows can cause irritability, poor concentration, a foggy head and depression.

Watch your table-salt intake. Use herbs to flavour your food.

Snacks for busy moments
It's always a good idea to be prepared with a healthy snack if you are on the run or at work. You could make your own trail mix from goji berries, cacao nibs, almonds, hazelnuts and pumpkin seeds. This will supply you with the minerals zinc and magnesium as well as B vitamins needed for energy. Or forget making anything and pick up a bag of unsalted almonds at a health-food store. Almonds have a proven cholesterol-lowering effect, have been found to be useful for weight loss as they provide a feeling of satiety and are an easy on-the-run snack to keep cravings in check.

My favourite way to deal with snacking when I am busy is to chuck an avocado, the perfect fast food, in my handbag. When I get to work, I slice the avocado in half and scoop out the avocado flesh with a spoon. Delicious!

Supplement and herb tips

Always consult your medical doctor before taking supplements and check with a herblist for the correct dosage of herbs. The following nutrients are helpful in supporting your adrenal glands: vitamins B5, B6, B12, C, pantothenic acid, magnesium, folic acid, zinc and essential fatty acids.

Adaptogenic herbs can help the body to adapt to stressful situations. Adaptogenic herbs include Rhodiola rosea, Siberian ginseng and Indian gooseberry or Amla. These have all been found to have antioxidant properties which is helpful given the increased potential for oxidative damage during stressful times.

Astragalus has been shown to improve spatial learning and memory and to reduce anxiety during times of stress.

Vitamin C may be used by the adrenal glands as part of the stress response. Extra vitamin C may be beneficial to stressed individuals.

The herb lemon balm (*Melissa officinalis* L.) has been found to have anti-anxiety effects.

General lifestyle tips

- Exercise is a proven stress reliever. Think about it: when have you ever been for a walk, jog, cycle or even just had a dance around the kitchen and *not* felt better for it?

- Yoga, visualization and meditation can all be beneficial for stress relief. And investigate Eastern disciplines like t'ai chi and chi gung.

- Make time for friends and family – it's easy to lose touch when you're working hard or feeling down. But having people to talk to and laugh with is key.

- Prioritize sleep – create a dark, welcoming bedroom environment, don't eat too late at night and don't watch TV or surf the internet or, worse, work in the hours leading up to bedtime. Get to bed at the same time every night if possible and make it early. Aim for ten o'clock.

- Find something that helps you to de-stress and include it weekly. It could be massage, reflexology, painting, visiting the cinema . . . whatever works for you.

Thrush

About half of all women will have thrush at some point in their lives, some experiencing regular bouts – it's an extremely common condition. It's an infection usually caused by the yeast *Candida albicans* but there are other types of candida that can cause it. Thrush mainly affects the vagina and surrounding area (although it occasionally occurs in the mouth). Candida occurs naturally in the gut, on the skin and in the vagina in balance with other beneficial bacteria which keep it in check. But if something upsets this balance and there's an overgrowth of candida, symptoms may arise.

These are typically vaginal soreness and itching, which is worse after sex. There's usually a thick, white, sticky discharge that may have a musty or yeasty smell. The genital area may be red and swollen and you may have pain during sex.

Triggers for an overgrowth of candida may include:

- Use of antibiotics
- Use of the contraceptive pill, HRT or an IUD
- A diet high in sugar and refined carbohydrates
- High alcohol intake
- Sex with an infected person
- Over-washing of the vagina or using scented products
- Pregnancy
- Diabetes
- Wearing synthetic underwear or tights

What you can do

You can buy creams, oral tablets and pessaries at the chemist to deal with a bout of thrush – although the cream can be effective in reducing itching, it's not a treatment on its own and you need to treat the infection inside the vagina. So a combination is best.

If symptoms don't clear up or keep coming back, see your doctor to ascertain whether your symptoms are actually caused by thrush or another infection (such as bacterial vaginosis, see page 130). Your GP can take a vaginal swab which is sent to the lab for testing.

Thrush often clears up on its own but it is important to encourage the growth of beneficial bacteria and change the vaginal and gut environment so that it is not so easy for yeast to thrive.

Gillian's diet tips

- Whole grains such as oats, quinoa, millet, buckwheat, brown rice and rye contain fibre needed for healthy bowel bacteria.

- Chicory and Jerusalem artichokes contain types of fibre that encourage the growth of good bacteria.

- Fresh fruit and vegetables are cleansing and immune-boosting.

- Garlic, onions, olive oil, chives, oregano, thyme and cinnamon all have antifungal properties.

- Drink pau d'arco tea for its ability to keep yeast levels in check.

- Steer clear of sugar, refined carbohydrates and alcohol as these may all encourage the yeast to thrive.

- Avoid yeast-based foods such as bread, buns and baked goods. Also avoid vinegar and other fermented foods.

Supplement and herb tips

Always consult your medical doctor before taking a course of supplements and check with a herbalist for the correct dosage of herbs.

- Acidophilus is a beneficial bacterium that should be present in the vagina and bowel to keep candida in check. Taking a daily supplement can help to re-establish healthy levels.

- Zinc is often low in women who get regular bouts of thrush. Pumpkin seeds, sesame seeds, seaweed, chicken, fish, brown rice, tahini are all sources of zinc but if you have thrush take a supplement, too.

- Take pau d'arco in tincture or capsule form.

- Caprylic acid can be an effective antifungal.

Beware candidiasis

Sometimes, an overgrowth of the intestinal yeast candida can become systemic and have a detrimental effect on your wellbeing as a whole. It's often triggered by stress, trauma or illness. Diagnosis is via blood, stool and other biochemical tests, and holistic treatment with diet and supplements is very effective. If you experience several of the following symptoms and can't figure out a cause, I'd urge you to see your GP, nutritionist, herbalist or homeopath and ask them to consider candidiasis:

- Allergies
- Athlete's foot
- Bloating
- Chronic fatigue
- Clogged sinuses
- Confusion (brain fog)
- Constipation
- Diarrhoea
- Digestive disturbances
- Easy bruising
- Excessive mucus
- Flaky skin
- Flatulence
- Food sensitivities
- Headaches/migraines
- Hypoglycaemia
  (low blood-sugar levels)
- Insomnia
- Joint/facial/ear pain
- Loss of libido
- Mucus in stools
- Nausea
- Night sweats
- Oedema (fluid retention)
- Persistent cough
- PMS
- Recurrent sinusitis
- Recurrent thrush
- Sensitivity to odours, fumes
- Sore, burning tongue
- Vaginal/anal itching

General lifestyle tips

- Apply calendula cream or gel to the irritated area around the vagina. Calendula has antifungal properties and helps to soothe irritation and itching.

- Insert live natural yoghurt into the vagina to help to encourage the growth of beneficial bacteria. Of course, eating natural yoghurt is a good idea if you don't fancy the insertion option.

- Pessaries containing acidophilus can also be used to re-populate the area with good bacteria.

- Bacteria thrive in warm, moist environments so avoid synthetic underwear and tights. Wear only natural fibres like cotton, hemp and silk which allow the skin to breathe and keep the area cool and dry.

- Tampons are often made from unnatural fibres that can cause irritation in the vagina. Try organic cotton-based sanitary towels or a moon cup instead. Or seek out organic, unbleached cotton tampons from your health-food store.

- Add five drops of lavender and three drops of tea tree essential oils to your bath. Both antifungals, they can help to reduce any infection that may be present.

- Use natural products for washing and on the skin. Avoid using scented bubble baths, douches, shower gels or applying any products to the vaginal area.

- Don't have sex until your thrush has cleared up. If you keep getting it, you and your partner may be passing it back and forth to each other, so your partner should be treated, too.

Common health concerns in pregnancy

DO NOT TAKE ANY SUPPLEMENTS OR HERBS DURING PREGNANCY ITSELF WITHOUT THE APPROVAL OF YOUR MEDICAL DOCTOR AND/OR HEALTH PRACTITIONER.

Constipation

If you have difficulty moving your bowels and/or experience a slow passage of waste products through the bowels leading to infrequent or difficult bowel movements, then you are most likely constipated. You are not alone. It is one of the most common gastro-intestinal complaints. Women are more prone than men, often at certain times during their menstrual cycle and particularly when pregnant. This is due to the relaxing effect female hormones can have on your intestines. My advice here will be helpful whether you're pregnant or not.

A proper functioning bowel should empty out regularly, once to twice daily, without effort. Difficult bowel movements such as sitting on the toilet for ages, trying to force something out, dropping only hard, little 'rabbit pellets', a slow transit time or a full, uncomfortable feeling as if you haven't fully emptied your bowels are signs that you may be constipated.

Blocked bowels can be the start of a litany of both minor and major health problems ranging from bad breath, diverticulitis, body odour, coated tongue, bloating, gas, hernia, headaches and varicose veins. Having to strain on the loo puts you at risk of haemorrhoids (see page 182) and a weakened pelvic floor. However, most bowel problems can be eliminated if treated in time.

Apart from pregnancy hormones, constipation can be caused by:

- A poor diet with a lack of fibre
- Dehydration
- A sedentary lifestyle
- Resisting the urge to open your bowels when you need to
- Taking certain types of iron supplements
- Ageing – elderly people often suffer from sluggish bowels
- Some medications
- Nutrient deficiencies or imbalances
- Long-term use of laxatives
- Anorexia or eating disorders
- Stress and tension

What you can do

Diet and lifestyle changes will almost certainly deal with your constipation. However, you should always report any sudden and unusual changes in your bowel habits to your GP. Never ignore blood in your stools, severe abdominal pain or unexplained weight loss. If the following measures don't help, you may also need to see your GP for further investigations.

Gillian's diet tips

Drink a cup of warm water with some fresh lemon squeezed into it first thing every morning (and again about two hours before bedtime). It's very cleansing and gets the bowels moving. Follow this with a cup of nettle tea.

A fruit smoothie with a superfood powder added is a great way to start the day.

Include cauliflower, cabbage, sauerkraut, Brussels sprouts, broccoli and all dark green, mineral-rich, leafy vegetables,

sprouted seeds and raw shelled hemp seeds in your diet –
they're all good sources of fibre and are liver strengtheners.

- Pulses, soaked figs, soaked flaxseeds and prunes are good
  movers, too.

- Grind a tablespoon of flaxseeds and soak them for a few
  hours in a cup of water. Stir this mixture and drink it before
  meals to help to lubricate the bowels.

- Flaxseed tea is helpful for bowel lubrication. You can make
  this by soaking a tablespoon of flaxseeds in half a pint of hot
  water overnight. Warm this mixture, strain and drink it in
  the morning.

- Hydration is important to avoid being backed up! So drink at
  least two litres of fluids a day (still water, herbal teas, vegetable
  juices and pure fruit juices). Consuming high-fluid foods
  such as soups and stews can also help to hydrate the colon.

- Well-cooked whole grains contain fibre and are an excellent
  way of getting water into the colon. Cook grains such as
  quinoa, brown rice and millet in three times the amount of
  water with the lid on until all the water has been absorbed.

- Good herbal teas include nettle, horsetail, chamomile
  and mint.

- Make sure that you get enough roughage in your diet. So, lots
  of high-fibre foods in the form of fruits and vegetables, please.

- Eggs can be constipating for some people as they tend to bind
  the contents of the gut and slow their passage out of the body.

- Spicy foods, sugar, sweets, tea and coffee should also be
  avoided due to their irritating effect on the bowel wall.

Supplement and herb tips

Always consult your medical doctor before embarking on a course of supplements, especially if you are pregnant, and check with a herbalist for the correct dosage of herbs.

The mineral magnesium is important for both bowel regularity and liver function, so a daily supplement may help.

Slippery elm powder in between meals is most helpful as it coats the walls of the intestines, easing the passage of wastes out of the body, and is not unpleasant in taste, so no excuses for you there.

IF YOU ARE NOT PREGNANT OR NOT TRYING TO BECOME PREGNANT, THE FOLLOWING MAY BE HELPFUL:

In cases of chronic constipation (but not if you are pregnant), use the following nutrients for the first three weeks: aloe vera, triphala, wild blue-green algae or spirulina, red chrysanthemum flower essence, flax oil, psyllium, milk thistle, vitamin C with bioflavanoids, vitamin B complex (rice-based), magnesium. Stronger herbs: turkey rhubarb and cascara sagrada will surely get things going in the right direction but should not be relied upon in the long term. You can often find these herbs in bowel formulas in health stores.

After three weeks you may wish to gradually reduce the amounts, and when the constipation clears you can discontinue this programme.

To maintain healthy bowel function and prevent sluggishness in future, beneficial bacteria in the form of acidophilus may help as well as a digestive enzyme complex with every meal. Include linseeds, pumpkin seeds and black sesame seeds in your diet.

General lifestyle tips

- If you want to get your bowels moving – get moving! Exercise will help your body to operate at its optimum level and some people find that it can help get a sluggish system moving.

- Slow down your eating habits. Chew your food thoroughly. I believe good digestion starts in the mouth. So I don't want to see you wolf your food down. You are not a vacuum cleaner and you are not in a race. Also, it's not nice to watch a person shovelling food down like there's no tomorrow.

- Don't ignore the need to go to the loo. I know some people have hang-ups about not going anywhere but their own bathroom, but if you need to go, *go*! Not responding to your body's natural signals can eventually have a negative effect on your normal bowel reflexes.

- Invest in a small stool approximately a foot high (a yoga stool or the type toddlers use to reach the loo is ideal). Place the stool in front of the toilet. When you sit on the toilet, place your feet on the stool. No, I'm not joking – I'm absolutely serious when I say that this will help you. The stool positions your body into more of a squatting position, improving bowel movements. Using a stool improves the angle of the rectum in the pelvis, making it easier to pass stools.

- Drink plenty of fluid. Not too much or you will feel bloated. Between eight and ten mugfuls a day is about right.

- Avoid alcohol, regular tea, coffee and cola as they are dehydrating.

- Avoid constipating medicines unless prescribed by your medical doctor.

Practise squatting. My clients swear by it! So on you go, ten squats on the double!

Massage the bowel in a circular, clockwise direction from the lower right side of the abdomen just above the right hip bone, up to just below the right rib cage, across the top of the abdomen and down to the left hip bone.

Reflexology can help some people. You can even do your own home treatment by massaging the arches of your feet in a clockwise direction. Even better, get your partner or friend to do it for you!

Gestational diabetes

Diabetes is caused by a lack of insulin, or insulin not working as it should, meaning your blood glucose levels become too high. For more about diabetes in general, see page 244.

During pregnancy, hormones block some of the usual actions of insulin in order to allow the baby to get sufficient glucose. So, coupled with the growth demands of the baby, a pregnant woman needs to produce quite a lot more insulin than normal. If your body cannot cope with the extra demands of pregnancy, gestational diabetes – a temporary form of the condition – may result. About one in 400 pregnant women develops gestational diabetes.

It usually arises in the second half of pregnancy and disappears once the baby is born. However, some people continue to be diabetic after the birth (it's also possible they were diabetic before the pregnancy but it went undiagnosed).

If you're expecting a baby, you'll have urine tests at all your antenatal appointments to check for protein (a sign of pre-eclampsia, see page 199) and glucose. This is not, however, the most reliable sign of diabetes so blood tests are also carried out. If you have raised blood glucose you'll be advised to have a glucose tolerance test which can give a firm diagnosis. You may not have experienced any symptoms, but possible signs include increased thirst, increased urination and tiredness – all common in pregnancy anyhow so hard to spot!

The reason gestational diabetes must be addressed is it may put you at higher risk of:

- Pre-eclampsia, which causes high blood pressure in pregnancy (see page 199)
- Premature labour
- A larger baby and more difficult delivery, with increased likelihood of a Caesarean
- Being advised to have an induced birth before full term
- Excess amniotic fluid
- Type 2 diabetes in later life (see page 244)

Your baby may have low blood sugar or jaundice after birth – both minor issues which usually correct themselves. There is also an increased risk of your baby being born with heart defects or respiratory problems.

There are certain risk factors for developing gestational diabetes. They include:

- A family history of gestational diabetes or diabetes
- Having previously had a large baby (over 4.5kg or 9lb 14oz)
- A previous stillbirth
- Being overweight
- Being an older mother
- Family origin – if you are a member of an ethnic group with a higher rate of type 2 diabetes

What you can do

If you suspect gestational diabetes, make an appointment to see your GP or midwife. It's more likely, however, that it will just be picked up at a routine antenatal check when you have a blood test. Once diagnosed, you'll be advised to go for more frequent antenatal checks and may be shown how to test your own blood glucose levels daily. So long as you're able to control your blood-sugar levels, you should be able to have a normal birth at full term. This is normally done with diet and exercise. Occasionally, insulin or metformin (a drug that is designed to improve the cells' response to insulin) is needed.

Gillian's diet and lifestyle tips

- Read my general advice on diabetes (page 244), and do follow all the dietary advice (seek approval from your doctor before taking any supplements, though).

- Eat small regular meals and snacks.

- Avoid sugar, refined carbohydrates, alcohol and artificial sweeteners.

- Take moderate daily exercise such as walking, yoga or swimming.

- Get outside every day with some skin exposed. This is important as the body can make vitamin D from the action of sunlight on the skin. Vitamin D helps your body to use insulin effectively.

- It is advisable to breastfeed your baby within an hour of delivery if possible.

- It is common for your blood-sugar levels to fall after the birth. Your midwife and medical doctor should bear this in mind if you are taking insulin or metformin. You'll need another oral glucose tolerance test six to eight weeks after delivery and then annual testing.

- If you're still taking insulin or metformin while breast-feeding, you're likely to need a reduced dose – seek your doctor's advice.

- Because your risk of developing diabetes in later life is increased, it's important to continue following my diet and lifestyle advice even when your gestational diabetes has ended, as a preventative measure.

Haemorrhoids

Haemorrhoids – also known as piles – are basically varicose veins of the rectum and anus. Symptoms can range from a sore, itchy anus and blood on the paper when you wipe, to large, bluish, inflamed veins protruding from the anus and causing significant discomfort or pain.

Haemorrhoids usually occur when the blood in the veins around the rectum and anus stops flowing. Straining on the loo and constipation are the main cause. And although both men and women can suffer from piles, women are particularly prone during pregnancy. This is due to the extra pressure placed on your pelvic veins by the weight of your uterus plus increased levels of blood circulating through your body, hormones weakening your vein walls, and a susceptibility to constipation in pregnancy, and you can see why it's a common problem.

Other contributory factors may include:

- Bad eating habits
- Lack of fibre
- Too much coffee or alcohol
- Laxative use
- Lack of exercise
- Sitting or standing for long periods of time
- Obesity
- Insufficient fluid intake
- Weak vein walls
- Heavy lifting or incorrect lifting technique
- Heredity: some people inherit a weakness of the vein walls in the anus
- Ageing

What you can do

The best way to avoid piles is to avoid constipation and straining on the toilet. Also follow my advice on page 174. If you're in discomfort, you may need a cream or suppositories from your chemist or health-food store (try the homeopathic alternatives). In more severe cases, you may need to see your GP for medication, injection or surgery. There is a range of removal processes depending on the severity of the condition.

As with constipation, always report any sudden and unusual changes in your bowel habits to your GP. Never ignore blood in your stools, severe abdominal or rectal pain or unexplained weight loss.

Gillian's diet tips

- Berries and cherries contain proanthocyanidins which can help to strengthen and heal capillary walls, so they're more resistant to piles. You can use berries in juices and smoothies, too.

- Buckwheat contains rutin which is also good for strengthening capillary walls.

- Include natural yoghurt for its gut-friendly probiotic properties. The beneficial bacteria in yoghurt can help to improve bowel function.

- Make sure your diet contains sufficient oils. The essential fats found in hemp, flax and pumpkin seeds and oils have an anti-inflammatory and healing effect.

- Dark green, leafy vegetables and alfalfa are sources of vitamin K, a good preventative.

- Avoid coffee, alcohol, junk food and sugar. They can cause dehydration which may lead to constipation and haemorrhoids.

- Get more fibre into your diet. So, lots of fruits and vegetables, please.

- Whole grains such as brown rice, quinoa, oats and millet are all excellent sources of fibre which is essential in preventing constipation.

- Drink plenty of water and herbal teas throughout the day. Warm fluids tend to be kinder on the digestive tract than very cold fluids.

Supplement and herb tips if you are NOT PREGNANT

Haemorrhoids can occur at any life stage. If you are NOT pregnant, here are my recommended supplements and herb tips. Always check with a herbalist for the correct dosage and combination and consult your doctor before embarking on a course of supplements.

- The herb bilberry is high in bioflavanoids which are anti-inflammatory compounds. Bioflavanoids help to relieve the distended veins of haemorrhoids.

- Take milk thistle to help soften the stool.

- The herb plantain can also help soften the stools and make them easier to pass.

- Butcher's broom can improve vein tone by reducing the inflammation of the tissue surrounding the haemorrhoid.

- Horse chestnut is also helpful for veins. It's available from health-food stores. You can also find it in homeopathic/herbal tinctures and creams for varicose veins and piles.

- B vitamins are essential for liver health and haemorrhoid-prone individuals are often low in the vital Bs. So take a daily B complex with extra B6.

- Vitamin E is healing and anti-inflammatory. You can take it internally and pierce open a capsule to apply it topically to reduce irritation and inflammation.

- Magnesium helps to relax the bowel and can help to get the bowels moving. Only take a small amount for a short period of time. And check first with your medical doctor.

General lifestyle tips

- If you have piles, sitting in a small basin of cold water offers relief by reducing inflammation and easing the engorged blood vessels. A sandwich bag filled with frozen peas or an ice pack are good alternatives.

- You can buy small cushioned or inflatable rings to make sitting more comfortable.

- Apply green clay which you will find in herbal or health-food stores. Mix it with water. It's messy, but may relieve the swelling and pain. To remove the clay, take a bath or shower. Witch-hazel compresses are good, too. To make a compress, simply soak a clean cloth (such as a hankie or flannel or a cotton pad) in a bowl of distilled witch hazel, wring out and hold it against the haemorrhoid for five minutes.

- Aloe vera can be applied topically for its healing effects. If you have an aloe vera plant, just break open a leaf and apply the gel to the affected area. Otherwise, you can buy pure aloe vera gel (available in health-food stores) to apply topically.

- Don't strain on the toilet. This will only make matters worse. See my advice on constipation (page 174) for how to use a foot stool when you use the loo. Eventually, after practising with the stool, you may even be able to get your feet up on the loo seat itself.

- Learn to lift correctly. Bend at your knees rather than your back. Breathe fully and let your legs take the strain.

- Warm (not hot) baths with essential oils can help to reduce any swelling and pain. Try adding a few drops of lavender oil to the bath water and relax for fifteen to twenty minutes. Do not use essential oils if pregnant.

Miscarriage

Miscarriage is the spontaneous loss of a pregnancy in the first twenty-four weeks. It's one of the most heartbreaking things that can happen to a woman and her partner. Sadly, it's common – it is thought as many as one in five pregnancies may end in miscarriage, most within the first twelve weeks. It is likely that many women have miscarriages without being aware of having been pregnant. The vast majority go on to have successful pregnancies in the future.

Many miscarriages happen without any known cause. Often the body is trying to make sure you have a baby that will have the best chance of surviving once born. It is thought that about half of all miscarriages are due to chromosomal defects caused by faulty cell division at the beginning of the pregnancy. Age is also a major factor – being over thirty-five makes miscarriage more likely. Other possible causes include:

- Fever from an infection
- High blood pressure
- Structural problems in the uterus or cervix
- Problems with the immune system with antibodies in the blood
- Smoking and alcohol
- Thyroid disorder

What you can do

- Follow the guidelines for pre-conceptual care before you get pregnant if possible (see page 98). Follow the guidelines for pregnancy once you have conceived (see page 107). Being well nourished is one of the best ways of ensuring a healthy pregnancy and a healthy baby.

- If you smoke, stop immediately.

- Avoid alcohol.

- Avoid unpasteurized milk and cheeses, raw honey, pâté and improperly cooked meals – these may contain bacteria that could lead to infection and illness.

- Avoid going on holiday to malaria areas.

- Take regular, moderate exercise.

- Start taking folic acid if you're planning to become pregnant or a multivitamin and mineral supplement designed for preconceptual or ante-natal care.

- In women with a history of miscarriage there may be a deficiency of the mineral manganese, so you may want to seek advice about supplementing for a short period with this important mineral. Every woman who has ever come to me with a history of miscarriage has tested deficient in this mineral.

'What could be better for the soul than taking five minutes to sit on a park bench, breathe deeply and feel the sun on your face?'

Morning sickness

About half of all pregnant women experience sickness or nausea in the second and third months of pregnancy. You won't usually experience it before the fourth week of pregnancy and it usually does not continue past the sixteenth. However, it is not limited to the morning and, unfortunately, for some women it continues throughout the pregnancy. Symptoms, as you'd expect, include nausea and often vomiting. This can make eating a healthy diet difficult at a time when it is most important to do so – which in itself can be a source of stress. Possible causes include:

- Vitamin deficiencies, especially B6
- High levels of pregnancy hormones
- Carrying twins or higher multiples – so higher levels of pregnancy hormones
- Tiredness and anxiety
- Rich, fried or fatty foods
- Hunger

What you can do

If you haven't been able to keep anything down for twenty-four hours, including fluids, you may have a condition called hyperemesis gravidarum which causes excessive vomiting in pregnancy. It is vital that you see your medical doctor if this is the case in order to avoid complications. Also see a medical doctor if the sickness persists past your fourteenth week of pregnancy or if you vomit blood.

Otherwise, it's simply a case of riding out the nausea until it subsides – it may only last a few days or weeks. The good news is that most women find something that works for them.

Gillian's diet tips

Unusual as it might sound, a common 'cure' for morning sickness is . . . eating! Low blood sugar is one of the main triggers so for many women coping with the symptoms is simply a case of getting used to eating more often. You need to eat small meals and snacks regularly throughout pregnancy – every two to three hours. Always keep some healthy snack foods with you. Fruit, nuts, seeds, avocados and whole grain crackers can all be life-savers. Don't let yourself get really hungry. Have a small snack before you go to bed to reduce the likelihood of waking in the night with nausea.

Foods rich in vitamin B6 may be helpful. These include eggs, spinach, fish, chicken, turkey, green vegetables, sunflower seeds, brown rice and bananas.

Peppermint and chamomile herbal teas can also be calming to the digestive tract.

Snacking on oat cakes or rye crackers may help to stave off nausea. If you suffer with sickness on rising in the morning, keep a snack by your bed to nibble before you get up and take your time over it. Getting out of bed with low blood sugar may trigger the sickness. A few nuts or seeds or a piece of fruit are also good options.

Most women find they favour bland foods over strong, rich-flavoured foods. Cooked whole grains such as brown rice, oats and quinoa are ideal.

It is vital to keep well hydrated, especially if you experience vomiting, so try to sip water throughout the day as much as you can. Barley water can be very soothing and nourishing. You can make it by simmering a handful of pot barley in five cups of water for twenty minutes. Strain and drink it throughout the day. You can add a squeeze of lemon juice if you like as well.

- Drink freshly pressed organic vegetable juices. These can replace minerals that may be lost through vomiting. They also supply readily available nutrients needed for your health and the foetal development.

- Avoid sugar and refined carbohydrates (they'll upset blood-sugar levels), alcohol, spices, caffeine and fatty foods.

- Pregnant women tend to have very strong instincts about what they need to eat. Listen to these instincts (unless they are telling you to eat lots of sugar or junk foods!).

Supplement and herb tips

- Although ginger is famous for its anti-nausea effects, I have not been able to find many women who believe that it has worked for them. Do **not** take ginger or ginger root capsules or essential oil while pregnant as ginger is what's called an emmenagogue which means that it tones reproductive organs and menstrual flow. So in HIGH dosages it could trigger a miscarriage early in pregnancy. Also, ginger has a cholagogue effect. This means that the properties within ginger promote the flow and discharge of bile into the duodenum by contracting the bile ducts. Cholagogues can stimulate contractions in the bowel. Any strong bowel contractions are contraindicated during the first trimester and it may stimulate a miscarriage.

General lifestyle tips

- Getting adequate sleep and rest is important. Having a nap or a rest during the day can be helpful.

- Avoid wearing clothes that are tight round the middle.

- Pregnant women have a heightened sense of smell and strong smells can trigger nausea. So avoid strong smells such as engine oil, cleaning products, perfumes, pungent foods or anything that makes you feel queasy.

- Breathe fully. Inhale into the diaphragm and exhale completely.

- Some women get good results from acupressure. Look for specially designed bands in the chemist or health-food store that put pressure on an acupuncture point on the underside of your wrist. (They're often marketed for travel sickness.) You can also stimulate this point yourself: measure three-finger widths from your wrist crease line. Press on the hollow between the tendons and you will experience a slight tenderness. Press the point firmly with your thumb as you exhale and release the pressure slightly when you inhale. Continue for a few minutes.

Post-natal depression

Pregnancy, childbirth and early motherhood are times of incredible change for women – physically, emotionally and socially. It's not surprising that, for some, issues with mental health can arise.

It's estimated that one in ten new mothers suffer from post-natal depression (PND) and 50–80 per cent will experience some form of baby blues – a shorter-lived, milder version. What's less well known (and less well diagnosed) is that 30–40 per cent may also experience episodes of depression and anxiety during pregnancy – called antenatal or perinatal depression.

It's normal to have mixed feelings about being pregnant, to worry about the future or sometimes feel down. Your moods will also fluctuate thanks to the changes in hormones. But if your depression or anxiety is more severe, affecting your daily life and ability to sleep, and making you overly tearful, lose your appetite or have obsessive thoughts or behaviour, speak to your midwife or medical doctor as soon as possible. Antenatal depression is more likely if you have a history of depression, miscarriage or loss, if you're under stress in your relationship or if yours is a higher-risk pregnancy.

Then there are the baby blues. Thanks to hormone changes immediately after birth, it's common to feel very tired, low and tearful, irritable or just extra sensitive to anything from a couple of days to a fortnight. Mothers often feel guilty because this is a time when they're supposed to be happiest. But the baby blues are natural and will lift.

Post-natal depression itself can be characterized by excessive anxiety about your baby and your ability to look after it, or perhaps the opposite – you have negative feelings about your baby and motherhood and are finding it hard to bond. You may even have disturbing thoughts about harming the baby. It may be a more extreme case of the baby blues that refuses to lift. PND is more likely if you have a personal or family history of depression, had a difficult birth or have had twins or higher multiple babies. It usually comes on within one to six months after the birth. If depressive feelings are affecting your daily life, are unusual for you and are affecting your ability to look after yourself and your baby, talk to your partner, family and friends and tell your health visitor or doctor as soon as possible.

The liver connection

It's my belief, based on years of experience in my practice and success with clients with PND, that the problem is less to do with simply being an emotional female and more biochemical. When a woman becomes pregnant, the liver has to process a bombardment of hormones. During and shortly after pregnancy, the mother's blood volume fluctuates massively. The liver is the key organ responsible for regulating, balancing, processing and handling such enormous and rapid biochemical changes to the mother's body, whether it be hormonal, blood or otherwise. If a new mum has feelings of sadness, confusion, anger or depression, additional excesses of hormones and adverse chemicals may be released. I have seen the up and down rollercoaster with more mothers than I care to count. And I'm pleased to report that working to support and nourish the liver gets amazing results. The liver connection that I talk about with post-natal depression is not recognized by Western medicine. However, it is an area that I like to address in my own practice.

What you can do

The most important thing, whatever type of depression you may be experiencing, is to try not to feel guilty – even though that emotion may be part and parcel of the condition itself! Many women are put off asking for help because they feel guilty that they're not enjoying pregnancy or motherhood more – or they're frightened their baby will be taken away from them. Rest assured this will not happen and health professionals are well trained to spot the signs and offer help and support. So, please, do ask for help.

In addition, try the following self-help measures to support your liver and balance your hormones.

Gillian's diet tips

- See my general advice on depression, page 346.

- Keeping blood-sugar levels balanced will help to prevent mood swings that will worsen symptoms. Eat little and often and see the section on mood swings, page 74.

- Certain fresh fruits help to stimulate energy flow through the liver, especially dark grapes, blackberries, huckleberries, strawberries, blueberries and raspberries.

- Sulphur-containing vegetables are high in specific liver-building enzymes. These include broccoli, cabbage, kale, kohlrabi, turnip roots and cauliflower.

- Eat foods which balance the flow of emotional and physical liver energy: grains, vegetables and legumes. Some of these foods when chewed thoroughly contain a healthy sweetness which is harmonizing to the liver. The natural inclination for a tired or stressed mum is to reach for a quick high-sugar fix – biscuits, cakes, ice cream, chocolate. When you feel that craving for a high-sugar fix coming on, train yourself to indulge in some of the following: amaranth, millet, quinoa, kidney beans, soya beans, tofu, peas, asparagus, basil, fennel, dill, cucumber, celery, mustard greens, seaweeds, radish leaves, romaine lettuce, watercress and red beets.

Veggie juices can be very revitalizing. Using a juicer, juice 6 carrots, 1 beetroot, 2 celery stalks and 1 apple together. It's tasty and very nourishing to the liver.

Supplement and herb tips

Always consult your medical doctor before embarking on a course of supplements and check with a herbalist for the correct dosage of herbs.

Folic acid

Essential fatty acids (take a fish oil or flaxseed supplement)

Zinc

Vitamin B complex with added B6

L-tyrosine

Blue-green algae supplement

Amino acid complex

There are many plants that can positively influence the liver's function. I have seen particularly excellent results in new mothers using the herbal plant silymarin, also called milk thistle. Silymarin contains flavonoid compounds which are antioxidant plant pigments. It protects the liver from damage, enhances the flow of bile and fats to and from the liver, and improves the detoxification process.

The following herbs may all be useful – try one at a time to see which works for you, or take them in rotation. Seek advice from a medical practitioner and herbalist first if you're breast-feeding. For example, you may need to take agnus castus for approximately three months to see a change.

- Agnus castus may help to balance female hormones.
- Rhodiola may support the adrenals and improve energy.
- Avena sativa (oat seeds) may be relaxing and useful if anxiety is a problem.
- Borage (starflower oil) may help to support the menstrual cycle.
- Siberian ginseng may help to adapt to stressors.
- Herbal teas of dandelion, nettle and red clover may be nourishing to the system.

General lifestyle tips

- The homeopathic remedies Kali Phos, Pulsatilla, Apis Mel, Nat Mur and Sepia may be helpful. For best results, see a homeopathic doctor.
- Bach flower remedies are very useful for emotional disorders and, like homeopathy, have no side effects and are completely safe for you and your baby (if breastfeeding). Walnut, Sweet Chestnut, Mustard and Gorse may all be helpful. Try Rescue Remedy, too, if you're feeling anxious.
- Your midwife, health visitor or GP can refer you for counselling. Don't be afraid to insist if you feel your concerns aren't being taken seriously.

- Say yes to all help offered by friends and family – particularly help with household chores and cooking so you have more time to spend bonding with your baby.

- Don't be afraid to leave the baby with his/her dad or other family member you trust so that you can get out of the house. Being depended on twenty-four/seven by this new life can feel overwhelming and some space can give you perspective.

- A recent study found mums of twins or multiples were far less likely to experience PND if they received antenatal classes specific to multiple births and tailored advice on parenting multiples. Speak to your midwife about what services are on offer.

- Studies have shown attending baby massage classes can help with difficulties in bonding with your baby and significantly reduce PND.

- Some osteopaths suggest that post-natal depression is linked to a downward placement of the uterus, resulting in a connecting pressure on the pituitary gland via the dura. It is well worth having this potential displacement checked.

'The energy of love is the most healing element in our existence.'

Pre-eclampsia

Pre-eclampsia only occurs in pregnancy, and usually late on during the second half of pregnancy. About one in ten women develop it. It's characterized by high blood pressure, protein in the urine and swelling (oedema) in the hands and feet. Left unchecked, blood pressure may continue to rise and you can add headaches, blurred vision and perhaps vomiting or pain in the upper abdomen to the list of symptoms.

The condition is thought to be caused by the blood vessels in the placenta not developing properly. This affects the delivery of oxygen and nutrients to the baby. The biggest danger, however, is if pre-eclampsia goes on to become eclampsia – a type of seizure that's fatal for about 2 per cent of mothers and 50 per cent of babies. Other complications of pre-eclampsia are rare but may include:

- Blood clotting which may lead to stroke
- Elevated liver enzymes and low platelet count meaning you are at risk of serious bleeding
- A smaller baby due to the reduced amount of oxygen and nutrients getting to the foetus
- Increased risk of stillbirth

To minimize the risk of pre-eclampsia, your blood pressure and proteins are monitored throughout pregnancy at your antenatal appointments. You may also be put under specialist care if you have a previous history of pre-eclampsia or a family history of the disease, high blood pressure before pregnancy, diabetes, systemic lupus erythematosus (SLE) or kidney disease, are obese, over forty or expecting twins or multiples. If you have a combination of high blood pressure and protein in your urine at any point, pre-eclampsia will be diagnosed. Bed rest is often prescribed to try to lower blood pressure and you may be admitted to hospital. Early delivery by inducing or Caesarean section is often advised and medications may be recommended to reduce complications. Once the baby and placenta have been delivered, pre-eclampsia tends to diminish. Magnesium sulphate may be administered via a drip in severe cases. Magnesium is relaxing and has an anticonvulsant effect.

What you can do

Avoiding the condition in the first place by maintaining a healthy blood pressure is the aim. Stress raises your blood pressure and challenges the body in many ways so it's important to get plenty of rest and relaxation. Reducing your stress levels while pregnant can help to lower your blood pressure. Although this won't necessarily prevent pre-eclampsia, your body will be in a much healthier condition and you will feel far more relaxed. Learn to manage stress with meditation, t'ai chi or breathing exercises, or find an antenatal yoga or Pilates class. Talk to your employer, partner, family, friends and midwife – or anyone else who might be able to help you address rising stress levels. Always report swollen hands or feet or other symptoms described above to your doctor or midwife immediately.

Gillian's diet and supplement tips

Always consult your medical doctor before embarking on
a course of supplements and check with a herbalist for the
correct dosage of herbs.

- Reduce your salt intake as excess sodium can increase
blood pressure.

- Eat plenty of fruit and vegetables. Aim for eight servings a
day. These are high in potassium needed to balance sodium,
as well as antioxidants which reduce free radical damage.
Several studies have shown a link between low levels of
antioxidants and increased risk of pre-eclampsia.

- In 1999 *The Lancet* published results of a trial in which
pregnant women with a history of pre-eclampsia or
abnormal blood flow to the placenta were given supplements
of the antioxidant vitamins C and E. The supplements
reduced the incidence of the condition by 76 per cent.

- Being deficient in calcium may increase your risk of
developing pre-eclampsia. Eat calcium-rich foods such as
green vegetables, almonds, tahini, chickpeas, haricot beans
and hazelnuts and consider a calcium supplement if you're
at risk.

- Eat a diet rich in fruit and vegetables, whole grains and
pulses.

- Magnesium may also be effective against pre-eclampsia
and works well with calcium.

- Take a daily multivitamin and mineral formula designed
for use in pregnancy.

Varicose veins

Varicose veins are enlarged, twisted, bulging veins, usually in your legs. At best, they can be unsightly, at worst they'll cause aching, itching, discomfort and can lead to eczema and leg ulcers.

They develop due to the improper functioning of the tiny one-way valves located in venous walls which help to transport the circulating blood back to the heart. If the valves are not working efficiently, blood can flow backwards and pool, causing superficial veins to swell and become visible through your skin.

One in four women will get varicose veins in their lifetime – more than double the rate in men. Like haemorrhoids (see page 182) varicose veins all too frequently form during or just after pregnancy. This is due to a combination of the extra weight of the baby putting pressure on your veins and pregnancy hormones relaxing the vein walls.

Other causes may include:

- Prolonged standing or sitting in the same position
- Lack of exercise
- A diet low in antioxidants, particularly vitamin C and bioflavanoids
- Being overweight or obese
- Age (the older you are, the more likely they'll occur)
- Genetic predisposition
- Sitting with crossed legs most of the time
- Weak vein walls
- Constipation

What you can do

Exercise is important, both for keeping your weight down and for promoting blood flow in the deep veins of your legs. Walking, swimming or anything else that works your calf muscles is particularly recommended. It's good to get moving even when you are pregnant but take it slowly – a gentle walk to get the blood circulating is sufficient. Stop if you feel out of breath or tired.

Try to avoid standing for long periods and when sitting don't cross your legs. Try to exercise your feet, ankles and calves as much as possible.

If varicose veins become a problem, do see your GP. They may need treatment with sclerotherapy (injections to close the faulty vein), or surgery to remove the vein. Laser surgery can work on more superficial 'thread' veins but not usually on varicose veins – it is more of a cosmetic than a medical treatment.

Gillian's diet tips

- Eat plenty of fibre and antioxidant-rich plant foods, which help to keep tissues strong and healthy.

- Fill up on foods high in vitamin C and bioflavonoids. Good food sources of both include citrus fruits, blackcurrants, grapes, cherries, apricots, rose hips, green peppers, tomatoes, broccoli and buckwheat groats. Buckwheat is particularly recommended for its rutin content. Rutin is a bioflavanoid that may help to strengthen the blood vessel walls.

- Omega-3 fats from fish oils or flaxseeds, hemp seeds and pumpkin seeds and their unrefined oils are anti-inflammatory and healing.

- Avoid processed foods, sugar, alcohol and caffeine.

Supplement and herb tips if you are NOT PREGNANT

The following supplement advice is only for women with varicose veins who are **not** pregnant. All herbs and supplements should be avoided when pregnant.

- Bilberry is the best herb to help varicose veins as it strengthens vein walls and capillaries.

- Nettle tea promotes venous elasticity. Alternate with dandelion and ginkgo biloba teas. Ginkgo biloba is good for improving circulation.

- Use tinctures of horsetail, a rich source of silica and bioflavanoids.

- Horse chestnut can be taken internally and applied externally to improve the health of the veins.

- Vitamin C and bioflavanoids are important for strengthening blood vessels so consider a supplement. Bioflavanoids also have the ability to regulate the permeability of blood capillaries. They stick to the collagen fibres in blood vessels, which restores the integrity of capillary walls.

- It's also worth supplementing with vitamin E, which may help to improve blood circulation and reduces pain and swelling.

- Vitamin B complex – the B vitamins aid healing.

- Lecithin helps to emulsify fats and aids healing.

- Co-enzyme Q10 may be helpful for circulation and cardiovascular health.

- An antioxidant formula that contains beta-carotene, selenium and zinc can aid healing and reduce inflammation.

If leg cramps are part of the problem, take magnesium to relax the muscles and nerves.

General lifestyle tips

Avoid sitting or standing for long periods of time. Move around as much as possible. Circle the feet and stretch the legs regularly.

Take exercise daily. Exercise is one of the best ways of getting the circulation going. Do not overdo it if pregnant. Gentle walking is fine. Always stop if you feel tired or out of breath.

Avoid socks or hosiery that have a tight band below the knee (such as pop socks).

Don't be scared of compression stockings or tights, especially during pregnancy. They help blood flow through veins more effectively, preventing and easing problems and can be claimed free on prescription during pregnancy. And these days they come in decent natural shades as well as fashionable opaque black – no more American-tan granny stockings!

Improve blood and lymph circulation and aid detoxification and exfoliation by dry-skin brushing before every bath or shower. Use a small, firm natural-bristle brush on a dry body. Start at the soles of the feet and work your way up the legs in long, brisk strokes; then up your arms and down your back. Always brush upwards towards the chest and avoid sensitive spots such as moles, warts and broken or bulging veins. Never use the brush on your face.

Avoid baths that are too hot. If you do bathe, add essential oils of rosemary or frankincense in the mornings; lavender, chamomile or rose at night. Do not use essential oils if pregnant as some have been linked to miscarriage. A weekly sea-salt bath is also soothing and relaxing.

- Massage the legs on a daily basis, working upwards towards your heart. Try making an aromatherapy massage oil to use when you do: add five drops each of lavender and cypress oils to 20ml sweet almond or grapeseed carrier oil. Again, do not use essential oils when pregnant.

- To help to ease varicose discomfort, a compress infused with horse-chestnut herb can be placed over the affected areas. Mix half a teaspoon of horse-chestnut powder with two cups of water and use it to soak a sterile cotton cloth. You can also buy gels or creams containing horse chestnut in your health-food store.

- Witch-hazel herb is another remedy that can be applied to the skin; a natural astringent, it tightens tissues and reduces pain.

- Calendula cream is healing and soothing.

- Do leg inversions as follows: lie on the floor on your back, placing your feet up onto a chair or couch or against the wall. Relax in this position for about fifteen minutes to improve circulation in your legs and aid blood flow back to the heart.

- Wear comfortable and roomy flat shoes rather than tight high heels. These are better for blood flow.

Dear Gillian,
I went to your website and signed up. Within a few days, my life was changed!!! I could eat a meal and not have tummy troubles. I had energy again, I didn't feel as achy and I had a positive attitude.

I have lost about 30 pounds since I did the questionnaire and still losing. I feel better, I exercise regularly now and my belly is flat instead of bloated.

Thank you!!!
Sylvia

Dear Gillian,
I'm only twenty-three, but I was having migraines, stomach pain and was very uncomfortable with my body. While I was in the normal range for my height (5ft 7in, 11stone 9lbs) my eating habits were not good. I would eat junk food and take-out late at night and pretty much starve all day. I didn't see anything wrong with it because I figured it was better than overeating. Now I know how wrong I was. Now I eat plenty of fruits and veggies as well as seeds and nuts. I'm glad that with your help I was able to correct my eating habits before it was too late. Now I have more energy, I'm happier and I have lost about 10lbs. Even my boyfriend is eating and feeling better. I plan on taking what you taught me and continuing this healthy path. Thank you for changing my life. I wish I could give you a big hug!! Thanks again!!
Kerry

Dear Gillian,
I am a thirty-seven-year-old woman who has struggled with weight and body image for most of my life. As a teenager I suffered from anorexia nervosa, and as an adult I have struggled to maintain a healthy weight and state of wellbeing.

I am writing to thank you for bringing information and guidelines about healthy eating to people like myself. Through watching and reading your philosophy, I have come to make healthy eating and exercise a value in my life. I no longer struggle with my weight going up and down, and I feel fantastic.

Thanks again for all you do to make us all brim with health!
Yours truly,
Claudia

Q: Dear Gillian,

I haven't felt like having sex since the birth of my first child, over a year ago. I really want to feel sexy but my body just won't let me. I love my husband, but it's starting to affect our relationship and intimacy. What's wrong with me?
  Susan, 32

A: Dear Susan,

First of all, please be reassured there's nothing wrong with you. Your predicament is very common. And, thankfully, there's a lot you can do to overcome it.

It is completely natural not to want to have sex after childbirth. If you are breastfeeding and looking after a baby already you simply may not feel like it. As your body recovers from childbirth and breastfeeding you will most probably find your desire for sex returns.

It may be that your usual female hormones haven't returned to pre-pregnancy levels. Herbs that may help to stimulate the ovarian hormones include damiana, gotu kola, motherwort and agnus castus.

It could also be that tiredness and stress have compromised the adrenal glands which are responsible for your zest for life and also partly for your sex hormones. If so, Siberian ginseng, rhodiola or ashwaghanda may be helpful. Yoga, t'ai chi, meditation and breathing exercises can all help to revitalize the adrenal glands.

Many women suffer from reduced thyroid hormone function after childbirth. Get your thyroid function tested. Kelp is an excellent source of iodine needed for thyroid hormones. Sprinkle a teaspoonful of kelp flakes onto soups or salads. Also eat two Brazil nuts a day to get the selenium needed for thyroid function.

If the problem is psychological in nature, for example on some level you may feel unattractive or you just don't like it, then counselling may be a good way forward. You may want to do this as an individual or as a couple. Do talk to your partner. Have a cuddle.

And are you eating properly? A lot of new mums do not eat well at all. In general, a healthy diet, regular but moderate exercise and relaxation promote many aspects of health. Going away on holiday and spending quality time with your partner can help you both remember how your relationship felt before the pregnancy and birth. Your old feelings for each other may well return.

Q: Dear Gillian,

I keep hearing about pelvic floor exercises – one friend tells me they make your sex life better, another said they stop you wetting yourself! What are they and should I be doing them?
  Sadie, 26

A: Dear Sadie,

I'm so glad you asked! It's never too early – or too late – to start exercising your pelvic floor muscles. And both your friends are right – there are myriad benefits to be gained from improving the tone of your pelvic floor.

  To locate your pelvic floor muscles, imagine you are trying to stop yourself from passing wind and stopping the flow of urine at the same time. The muscles that you use to do this are your pelvic floor muscles.

  Pelvic floor exercises are also called Kegel exercises. You can do them sitting or lying down. Breathe normally and pull up your pelvic floor muscles. Hold them for five seconds then relax the pelvic floor completely. Repeat this five times. You can gradually increase the length of time you hold your pelvic floor muscles up and the number of repetitions.

  Once you have got the hang of these, you can also try fast pelvic floor exercises. This involves pulling up your pelvic floor muscles and letting go very quickly. Repeat this ten times being sure to breathe while you are doing it. You should not be holding your breath, lifting your buttocks, holding in your tummy or squeezing your legs together while doing pelvic floor exercises. The movement is largely internal so you can do them while waiting for the bus or queuing up in the supermarket and no one need know!

  It's possible to get vaginal cones with which to practise your pelvic floor exercises. This involves inserting the cones into the vagina and contracting and relaxing as above. Some women find this easier but they are not strictly necessary. Talk to your GP if you want to try these.

  Improving the tone of your pelvic floor can make sex more enjoyable with stronger orgasms. Women with well-toned pelvic floor muscles often experience easier childbirth and a faster recovery from childbirth. If you keep the pelvic floor exercises up, you are likely to maintain good bladder control as you get older, too.

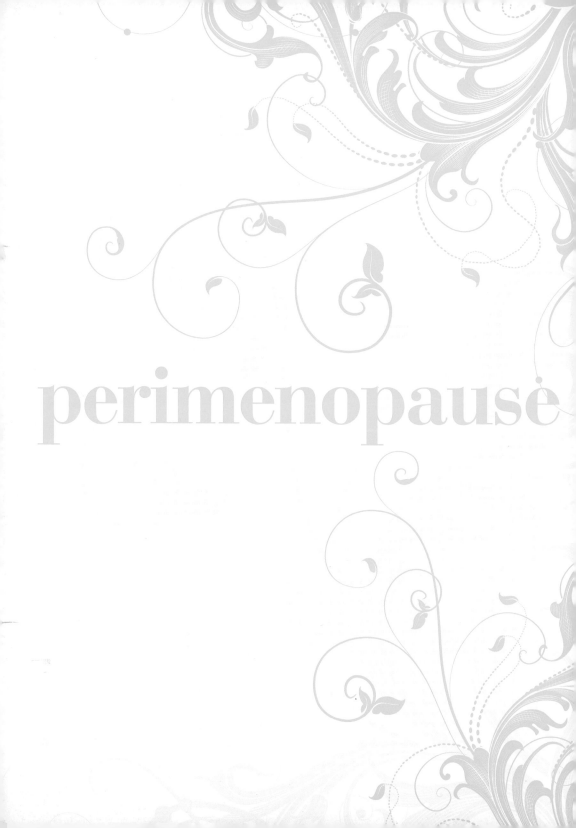

perimenopause

I'm fed up with the menopause getting such a bad rap! So many of my new clients seem to dread it, but I teach them there's nothing to fear. Far from a negative experience, this transition is a positive, liberating time. In some cultures, it's celebrated. And with the right action and attitude, it really can be a breeze.

Now in this section of the book, I use the word perimenopause. This refers to the years and months leading up to the menopause itself, which is actually just one event – your last-ever period.

If you're reading this and you're in your early forties or even late thirties you may be about to flick to another section, thinking, Well this clearly isn't for me . . . But hold your horses!

The fact is, while the average age for menopause itself in the UK is 51, the perimenopause can begin anything from a few years to a decade earlier. (A clue is to ask your mum when she had hers – if it was early or late, chances are you might just follow a similar pattern.) If you smoke, your menopause and so perimenopause will probably start a year or two earlier.

During these years, your oestrogen levels are on a fluctuating decline and this may (or may not) cause various symptoms. If you don't understand that these symptoms are down to your hormones, it can be a baffling and distressing time. So why stay in the dark? I'm here to enlighten you.

Like puberty, the perimenopause is not an overnight experience. What happens is your body's production of female hormones, oestrogen and progesterone, gradually wanes. As oestrogen production in particular falls, it triggers your brain to release higher quantities of other hormones (luteinizing hormone or LH, and follicle stimulating hormone, FSH) in an attempt to make your ovaries work harder. But still the number and quality of the eggs released from your ovaries inevitably falls and your fertility decreases.

Ultimately, of course, menopause marks the end of your reproductive years. But this is not something many women necessarily want to think about when they're in their early forties. These days, forty is younger than ever and lots of you are still raising families – even *starting* families – during this decade. So, believe me, I'm not about trying to make you feel old! You are most certainly still a young thing. I just believe it's useful to know what's going on in your body, so you can recognize and address any health niggles that may present themselves.

Early symptoms

The first signs that you may be entering perimenopause are likely to be mood swings and changes to your menstrual cycle. Your periods may start to become heavier, less regular, perhaps with longer gaps between them. Then they might return to normal for a few months. It can be a confusing time.

There's a myth that PMS worsens as you get older, because many women describe an increase in period problems, mood swings, skin problems and the like when they reach their forties. The reality is your hormones are fluctuating as they did during puberty, at the start of your reproductive life.

Many women find they experience unexplained weight gain, especially around the waist at this stage in their lives. Although this isn't thought to be directly related to the menopause, it is something that must be considered in this life stage. It is due to a combination of dwindling oestrogen and also a possible general slowing down of your metabolism as you age.

Later symptoms

As perimenopause progresses and you near menopause itself (and for a year or so afterwards), the other symptoms people think of as more 'typically menopausal' can occur. Remember I said *can* – this is by no means certain! They may include:

- Hot flushes
- Night sweats
- Even less frequent/more erratic periods
- Tiredness
- Depression
- Vaginal dryness
- Urinary tract infections (UTIs)
- Headaches
- Insomnia
- Joint pain
- Palpitations
- Low (or frustratingly high!) libido

I can't emphasize enough, however, that this needn't be your experience. The menopause is so often portrayed as a rotten time for women, when the reality can mean freedom, joy and sensuality. And even if you do come across some of these symptoms, I have a wealth of advice for you on how to prevent, limit or even eliminate them.

Hormone replacement therapy – my view

I am not in favour of hormone replacement therapy (HRT). As the controversy persists about its rights and wrongs, I try my best to convince women that the easiest way to ensure a smooth transition through menopause is by healthy living. Eating healthily and maintaining a good weight will help your body to best cope with the transition you are about to go through. In my practice, my perimenopausal patients never need HRT, since their hormones, glands and organs are so very balanced and in proper working order.

HRT usually involves tablets, ointments or patches that contain oestrogen or a combination of oestrogen and progesterone (called combined HRT). It's designed to counteract the effects of the natural reduction in oestrogen that women experience during the menopause. The word I would draw your attention to here is 'natural' – I don't believe we *need* to replace these hormones artificially, because they're *supposed* to be declining.

However, each woman must decide for herself whether she wants to take HRT or not, and it's important to make an informed decision.

Advantages of HRT

- Reduction in menopausal symptoms, such as mood disturbances, hot flushes, vaginal dryness and dry skin.

- Reduced risk of osteoporosis and non-vertebral fractures in post-menopausal women – this may be because oestrogen slows down the rate at which old bone is broken down.

- Possible reduced risk of colorectal cancer.

- Possible reduced risk of heart disease – if HRT is started at the onset of menopause while the arteries are still healthy, it may help to protect the cardiovascular system. But if women start HRT more than ten years after menopause, there is evidence to suggest it can increase the risk of heart disease.

Disadvantages of HRT

- There's growing evidence that HRT increases the risk of developing breast cancer, including research by Cancer Research UK and the Women's Health Initiative. It may be that HRT stimulates the growth of latent tumours or cancer cells which would not otherwise have become clinically significant. A Belgian study found that in areas where HRT use declined, so did the incidence of breast cancer. More research on the matter is ongoing. The risk is reduced within a few years of stopping HRT.

- Oestrogen-only HRT may increase the risk of endometrial cancer. However, if progesterone is also given, the risk is reduced.

- Long-term use of unopposed and combined HRT increases the risk of ovarian cancer. Stopping HRT reduces this risk.

- HRT may lead to increased weight and an increased waist-to-hip ratio – both of which can lead to an increased risk of cardiovascular disease and diabetes.

- The longer HRT is taken, the greater the risk of developing problems. Once you stop HRT, your risk of developing the above conditions decreases.

The choice is yours and not one I intend to get in the middle of. Make an informed choice. Get the facts under your belt and most definitely discuss the pros and cons with your GP who will be on the receiving end of the most up-to-date information on the topic. A good old chat with your GP about the issue will ensure that you are informed and comfortable with your choice on this matter.

'These days, forty is younger than ever and lots of you are still raising families – even starting families – during this decade.'

The importance of good nutrition

If you want to make the most of your forties and fifties, eating healthily and modifying your lifestyle is a *must*. I'm in no doubt whatsoever that it enables your body to adjust to the changes associated with perimenopause. The key areas you'll need to address during this time are:

Diet and hormone balance

Fluctuating hormones cause most of the symptoms of perimenopause. And while you can't change what nature is doing to your hormone levels, you can help to even out the peaks and troughs to give yourself an easier ride.

Diet-wise, any woman with signs of hormonal imbalance needs to consider three different hormone systems: blood-sugar hormones (insulin), adrenal hormones (stress and sex hormones) and ovarian hormones (sex hormones). You also need to look after your liver as it's responsible for processing hormones.

In the body, of course, all these hormone systems are interconnected and influence each other in countless ways. A healthy diet, regular exercise and stress management are the most beneficial, cost-effective and enjoyable ways of helping to prevent many of the conditions associated with menopause.

- Stabilize your blood-sugar levels by reducing the amount of sugar and refined foods you eat.

- It is my belief that eating plenty of phyto-oestrogen-rich fruit, veg, pulses and soya products – they have a hormone-balancing and mild oestrogenic effect – is helpful as your own levels of oestrogen start to decline (see 'The lowdown on phyto-oestrogens', page 229).

It may help to include foods high in the essential fatty acids. such as oily fish, nuts and seeds.

Weight gain

'Hang on a minute – where did my waist go?' This is a cry I often hear from women in their forties. They find it harder and harder to keep the weight off, and excess fat seems to settle around their middles. They may turn from 'pears' into 'apples'. Why?

During and directly after the menopause there is a tendency for some women to gain weight with a redistribution of body fat from the hips, buttocks and thighs to the abdomen. It is thought that oestrogen has a positive effect on fat deposition, directing it towards the breasts, hips and thighs (leading to the classic female pear shape). Once oestrogen levels start to decline this protective effect is lost and fat is deposited around the middle of the body leading to the less healthy apple shape.

I know, I know, it's unfair – I hear you! But you're going to have to be on your guard, because being overweight is a serious health risk. And abdominal fat, in particular, is a real baddie (see the section on metabolic syndrome, page 261). If you have a body mass index (BMI) of 25 or over, a waist measurement of 32in or more, or a waist-to-hip ratio of 0.8 or more (divide your waist measurement by your hip measurement), alarm bells should be ringing.

The bottom line is that unless you're genetically blessed with slimness, you have to watch your weight in your forties. Now this does not mean crash diets. It means exercising, eating healthily and being aware of the following food facts:

1   There is a link between abdominal weight gain, your blood-sugar control and insulin levels. When we eat carbohydrates these break down into glucose in the gut. Glucose enters the bloodstream, raising blood-sugar levels. Glucose provides vital fuel for the body, but we only need a small amount in the bloodstream at any one time. To keep blood-sugar levels on an even keel the pancreas releases the hormone insulin, to carry glucose from the blood to the liver and muscles where it can be stored as glycogen for energy requirements later on. Once glycogen stores become full, glucose can be converted to fat.

2   However, some folks can end up insulin-resistant. It's not actually known what causes insulin resistance, but it seems that some people's tissues stop responding to insulin. This means the body produces an increasing amount of insulin in order to bring blood-glucose levels down to a safe level. Still with me? Good! Now insulin is a storage hormone. The more you produce the more likely you are to convert glucose to fat which can lead to increased weight gain, most typically around your middle.

3   As with type-2 diabetes, people are developing insulin resistance at an increasingly younger age. Diets high in sugar, processed foods, alcohol and lack of exercise are contributory factors. Hence the increase in number of apple-shaped younger women.

4   Simple carbohydrates, found in sugary and refined foods, break down rapidly into glucose causing a blood-sugar spike and a rush of insulin. If you regularly consume simple carbs, you might just be looking at the result of these sugary binges on your belly! Steer clear of simple carbs. It's that simple!

- Avoid sugar in all forms.

- Avoid refined carbohydrates such as sugary breakfast cereals, white bread, baguettes, white pasta, white rice, crisps and pastries.

- Avoid alcohol, caffeine and nicotine – these are all stimulants that raise blood sugar.

- Eat small meals and snacks rather than large meals.

- Eat good quality protein – protein slows the breakdown of carbohydrates into glucose. Combine animal protein such as chicken or fish with vegetables and salads. Combine plant proteins (nuts, seeds, lentils, beans, soya) with grains and vegetables.

- Eat fibre with every meal – fibre is an indigestible carbohydrate that does not raise blood sugar or insulin but does slow carb breakdown. Fibre is found in lentils, beans, whole grains and vegetables.

- Get your bahookee moving! Exercise improves cellular response to insulin, helps to normalize appetite and, of course, burns off glucose and fat.

Top foods for your perimenopausal years

- **SOYA** This is a top-quality protein. Try tofu, tempeh, miso, natto. Avoid texturized vegetable protein and soya isolates.

- **FOODS RICH IN CALCIUM AND VITAMIN D** These help prevent osteoporosis and heart disease. (Vitamin D also comes from exposure to sunlight.)

ALMONDS These are rich in calcium and magnesium needed for bone health and cardiovascular health.

FLAXSEEDS As well as being a good source of omega-3 essential fats, these contain lignans that have phyto-oestrogenic effects once they've been metabolized by bacteria in the gut.

BEETROOT This vegetable is an excellent blood builder as well as being stimulating to the liver. A sluggish liver can greatly exacerbate symptoms and health problems.

SARDINES Canned fish with bones, such as sardines, provide lots of calcium as well the anti-inflammatory omega-3 fats that can help to reduce or prevent symptoms of hormonal imbalances.

GREEN VEGETABLES These provide calcium, magnesium and B vitamins, all needed for hormonal balance and bone health.

BROWN RICE An excellent source of fibre needed to remove old hormones and cholesterol from the body.

WHEATGERM A rich source of vitamin E which can help to reduce menopausal symptoms. Also needed for skin health and healing.

MUNG BEANS These are cooling and cleansing for the body and easy to digest.

PRUNES Famous for keeping bowels regular, prunes are also a rich source of antioxidants needed to protect the body from ageing and disease.

Top snacks

Dried apricots are rich in potassium needed for cardiovascular health and water balance. They are also high in iron which is often low at this time of life. Make sure you buy sulphur-free ones.

Sunflower seeds are rich in B vitamins needed for adrenal health and general hormone balance.

Toasted nori strips give you the iodine needed for thyroid health and metabolism.

Natural soya yoghurt is a good source of phyto-oestrogens, calcium and magnesium.

Goji berries are one of the best sources of antioxidants.

Hummous provides both protein and fibre (so is great for blood-sugar balance) as well as calcium and magnesium.

Foods to avoid

- Sugar will only upset your blood-sugar levels and increase your risk of weight gain and diabetes.

- Coffee acts as a stimulant, preventing the absorption of calcium which can contribute to osteoporosis.

- Processed meats (such as ham, sausages, salamis) are associated with many health problems that you become more susceptible to as time goes on, particularly bowel cancer.

- Red meat and dairy products contain potentially inflammatory saturated fats and have acid-forming properties. In order to neutralize the acid, minerals such as calcium are taken from body stores such as the bones and heart muscle, increasing your risk of osteoporosis.

- Hot spices, such as chilli peppers, can trigger hot flushes.

- Alcohol creates more work for your liver and provides empty calories. It ultimately acts as a depressant.

- Wheat is a source of gluten which is sticky and hard to digest. It often exacerbates digestive problems, weight problems and low moods.

'With the right action and attitude, it really can be a breeze.'

Food swaps

SWAP: Pasta carbonara
FOR: Wholemeal pasta with tuna and broccoli in a herb and tomato sauce

SWAP: Jacket potato with butter and cheese
FOR: Sweet potato with hummous and green salad

SWAP: Chicken and bacon Caesar salad
FOR: Grilled chicken with beetroot and tomato salad

SWAP: Breaded cod and chips
FOR: Grilled cod, baked sweet potato, steamed green beans and broccoli

SWAP: Cappuccino
FOR: Dandelion coffee with rice milk

Supplement and herb tips

Always consult your medical doctor before embarking on a course of supplements and check with a herbalist for the correct dosage of herbs.

- **CALCIUM** is a must to protect your bones. You'll also need vitamin D so that your body can utilize the calcium. Vitamin D mainly comes from the sun's contact with the skin.

- **VITAMIN C** with bioflavonoids has been shown to help to reduce hot flushes.

- **VITAMIN E** can also help to reduce hot flushes and vaginal dryness, and it's known to reduce heart-attack risk.

- **THE B VITAMINS** are known as mood vitamins and can reduce stress, anxiety, irritability, fatigue and poor concentration, giving the adrenals a rest. They may also help energy levels.

- **THE MINERAL MAGNESIUM** is known as 'nature's tranquillizer', because it alleviates symptoms such as anxiety and mood changes. It's also useful for bones.

- **DEHYDROEPIANDROSTERONE** (DHEA) is a hormone naturally produced in the body, and its levels tend to decline naturally with age. You can get a synthetic version of it on prescription which can help to increase oestrogen levels. If you're having a really bad time with menopause, ask your GP about this.

- **GAMMA ORYZANOL** is usually derived from rice bran oil and contains beneficial substances including sterols, ferulic acid and antioxidants. I have recommended it to many of my perimenopausal clients to positive effect.

AGNUS CASTUS, also known as vitex agnus castus and sometimes chaste berry, is my number one recommendation for my clients. It acts as an adaptogen, balancing female hormone production and thereby wiping out a wide range of symptoms.

BLACK COHOSH AND DONG QUAI can also help to restore hormonal balance and so ease symptoms, particularly hot flushes and vaginal dryness.

SAGE contains isoflavones, a type of phyto-oestrogen (see 'The lowdown on phyto-oestrogens', page 229). Its mild oestrogenic effect may alleviate hot flushes.

MILK THISTLE can be useful at menopause because it supports the liver and helps it to excrete old hormones and toxins.

GINKGO BILOBA has been shown to have a rejuvenating effect on the brain – it helps you to feel more 'with it'!

ANGELICA is well known as a tonic for the female reproductive system, regulating hormonal control and improving the rhythm of the menstrual cycle.

RED CLOVER is a good overall tonic; it is one of the more essential herbs for balancing hormones because of its high vitamin content. It is particularly high in B vitamins.

VALERIAN can help you to sleep without the side effects of orthodox drugs. Drink a cup of chamomile tea with a few drops of valerian tincture an hour before bed. Or try valerian tea.

(For more supplements to address specific ailments, see the Perimenopause conditions section, starting on page 242)

Feed your bones

By the age of thirty-five, your bone density will have peaked. Then, with the onset of perimenopause, you can no longer rely on the bone-protective effects of oestrogen and progesterone. Oestrogen reduces the breakdown of bone so I'd highly recommend reading the section on osteoporosis (page 387) as its dietary and exercise advice is pertinent to you now to prevent future problems. And you really need to make a conscious effort to ensure you eat more calcium-rich foods.

When you read the word calcium, dairy products like milk and cheese probably spring to mind. But not everyone does well with dairy. Many people are intolerant to it; it can be high in fat and difficult to digest for others. If you really want to drink cow's milk, please boil it first. This renders the molecules of the milk smaller and thus easier to digest. Bear in mind that cow's milk is low in magnesium. Yet calcium can only be efficiently absorbed alongside enough vitamin D, boron and magnesium. It's up to you, but I'd urge you to seek out as many additional sources of calcium as you can as well as sources of magnesium. Also, it is not so much the amount of calcium you take in that matters but the amount of that calcium that your body is able to absorb and utilize.

Here's some inspiration. Good non-dairy sources of calcium include: green vegetables (broccoli, savoy cabbage, kale, Brussel's sprouts, quinoa, cavolo nero, chicory, pak choi, romaine lettuce, salad leaves), canned fish with bones, almonds, sesame seeds, tahini, carob, dulse, figs, hazelnuts, alfalfa, kombu and wakame.

Sources of calcium

(mg of calcium per average serving)

Food	Serving size	mg of calcium
Cheddar cheese	25g	200mg
Cottage cheese	½ cup	65 mg
Natural yoghurt	100g	190mg
Goat's milk	240ml	326mg
Goat's cheese	25g	33mg
Watercress	1 cup	40mg
Sardines (canned with bones)	1 can	400mg
Tofu	100g	130mg
Broccoli (cooked)	1 cup	180mg
Kale (cooked)	½ cup	90mg
Sesame seeds	25g/1oz	280mg
Kombu (dried)	10g	70mg
Figs (dried)	½ cup	150mg
Almonds	25g/1oz	75mg
Chickpeas (cooked)	1 cup	75mg
White beans (cooked)	1 cup	140mg
Quinoa (cooked)	1 cup	35mg
Amaranth (cooked)	½ cup	135mg
Molasses	tbsp/15ml	150mg
Tahini	2 tbsp	130mg

The lowdown on phyto-oestrogens

You'll read the words 'phyto-oestrogen' and 'isoflavone' a lot in this section, as well as in anything on natural approaches to the menopause. So what are they?

Well, phyto-oestrogens are naturally occurring plant chemicals that have a mild oestrogenic-like action. They stimulate oestrogen receptors throughout the body, helping to balance hormone levels and ease menopausal symptoms. Phyto-oestrogens are part of a group of plant chemicals called isoflavones found in all fruit, vegetables and cereals (good sources include linseeds, whole grains, green veggies, garlic, fennel, celery, rhubarb, parsley and hops).

The four most beneficial oestrogenic isoflavones are called diadzen, genistein, formononetin and biochanin. They're found in legumes, such as soya beans, lentils, beans and chickpeas, as well as red clover leaves.

The Japanese diet is naturally much higher in phyto-oestrogens (up to thirty times higher, in fact), and the menopause simply isn't recognized in Japan in the same negative way as it often is in the West. Japanese women report fewer, if any, symptoms. Coincidence? I think not . . .

Phyto-oestrogens: a booster

Natural soya yoghurt with ground flaxseeds, almonds and wheatgerm is a great quick snack amd is packed with oestrogenic properties.

Tofu and vegetable satay skewers

SERVES 4-6

1 large red pepper, deseeded and cut into roughly 3cm pieces
1 large yellow pepper, deseeded and cut into roughly 3cm pieces
2 medium courgettes, trimmed and cut into roughly 1.5cm slices
24 button mushrooms, wiped
250g firm tofu, drained and patted dry with kitchen paper
  to remove excess water

For the marinade

2 large garlic cloves, peeled and crushed
1 1/2 tsp organic vegetable bouillon (stock) powder
2 tbsp agave syrup
1/2 tbsp ground coriander
1 tbsp ground cumin
1 1/2 tsp ground turmeric
100ml coconut milk

1 In a large glass bowl (it has to be glass as the turmeric may stain), mix together the marinade ingredients.

2 Cut the tofu into roughly 2.5cm cubes. Place in a medium glass bowl and spoon over just enough marinade to coat. Use a metal spoon to gently mix together, taking care not to break the tofu.

3 Add peppers, mushrooms and courgettes to the rest of the marinade and mix so everything is evenly coated. Cover both bowls with plastic film and leave to marinate in the fridge for at least 1 hour or overnight.

4 Using a disposable glove to protect your fingers from the turmeric, thread alternate pieces of vegetable and tofu onto metal or well-soaked bamboo skewers. Cook under a preheated hot grill or barbecue for 3-4 mins on each side until lightly browned and piping hot.

Soya bean and pea soup

SERVES 2
2 sachets miso soup or stock cubes
4 (40g) spring onions
2 celery sticks
125g frozen soya beans
125g frozen peas
Handful fresh mint leaves

1 Put on the kettle to boil. Place the miso soup in a medium-sized saucepan and pour 500ml boiling water into the pan.

2 Place pan over a high heat to bring the soup back to the boil. Meanwhile, finely slice the spring onion and celery, reserve the green top of the onion and a handful of celery to garnish. Add the onion and celery to the boiling stock.

3 Measure out the beans and peas and add them to the pan. Return the mixture to boiling point then add the mint. Cover the pan with a lid and leave to simmer for 4 minutes.

4 Remove from the heat and blend until smooth.

5 Spoon into 2 bowls and top with the spring onion tops and celery and serve.

Note: If you are using a glass blender, allow the mixture to cool slightly before blending.

Important lifestyle advice for perimenopause

Exercise

There is simply no way you can get away with not exercising in your perimenopausal years if you want to stay healthy. It's vital to keep your heart healthy, to keep your weight down, to boost your mood and to protect your bones. Exercise burns calories but, perhaps more importantly, it helps to maintain and build muscle. The more muscle you have, the higher your metabolic rate will be – in other words, you'll burn more calories, even at rest. The more muscle you have, the stronger you are and the better protected your skeleton – both because you're less likely to have an accident and because weight-bearing activity increases bone density so fractures are less likely.

You should aim for thirty minutes of moderate-intensity exercise a day. That's not a lazy stroll, that's a purposeful, brisk walk. Or it's a cycle, a swim, an aerobics or dance class. It's anything you love doing, but that gets you slightly sweating and out of breath (I know what you're thinking and, yes, sex counts!).

Using resistance bands, a weights machine or free weights at the gym, two or three times a week, gets you extra brownie points. And I can't recommend highly enough the muscle-building, posture-perfecting and stress-relieving benefits of yoga and Pilates.

Sleep

Disturbance to your normal sleep pattern can be one of the most frustrating symptoms of perimenopause. You may

How do I know when 'it's happened' and I'm post-menopausal?

It can be hard to know when you've actually 'gone through The Change', as they say – when you've experienced the menopause itself and your last-ever period has come and gone. If your periods have slowed right down, you may *think* they've stopped, then suddenly 'flow comes to town' again and catches you out (typically, on the day you choose to wear tight, white jeans . . .). For this reason, medical doctors will only diagnose you as having gone through the menopause in retrospect. That's why it's a good idea to keep a note of any periods or spotting you may have in your diary. You're medically classed as post-menopausal when your last period was a year or more ago. If you're really keen to know, you could ask your GP to run tests.

often be woken by hot flushes and night sweats, or just find you're generally sleepless (a partner's snoring doesn't help, either!). All the measures described in this section for balancing hormones will help, and see 'Hot flushes', page 256. Have a read, too, of my general advice on sleep patterns in the 'Post-menopause and beyond' section (page 304), as this applies to everyone.

I must point out, too, that a key reason for not sleeping well is lack of activity during the day. So now you have yet another reason to up your exercise levels – I will bet my last adzuki bean that if you add thirty minutes' more activity to your day, you'll sleep better that night.

Sex

You may have heard reports that women reach their sexual peak later in life than men. Well, I'm happy to confirm those reports! By your late thirties or early forties you're likely to experience an increase (sometimes quite intense) in libido. This is down to fluctuating hormone levels and possible changes in your menstrual cycle. Many women, however, experience the opposite and their libido falls.

As perimenopause goes on, production of the sex hormones – testosterone, oestrogen and progesterone – can become unpredictable. This affects different women in different ways, but it will most probably have some impact on your sex life. Whether you feel more or less sexual, remember there are no rights or wrongs and all levels of desire are normal. However, if you'd like to boost your sex drive, see 'Low libido', page 377.

One of the later symptoms of perimenopause can be vaginal thinning and dryness, which can affect your enjoyment of sex. For my advice, see page 281.

Health checks and tests

Although you won't yet be invited for mammograms on the NHS to check for breast cancer, it's vital to perform regular self-checks and be breast-aware (see the 'Post-menopause' section, page 309). You must also continue to attend your regular cervical smear tests when invited – make sure you're registered with a GP.

Your GP may also invite you for a vascular risk assessment, once you're over forty. This involves looking at your blood pressure, blood cholesterol, blood sugars, weight, family history and lifestyle (such as smoking history, diet and so on). The medical doctor can then work out your percentage risk of cardiovascular problems, such as heart disease, over the next ten years. If you're not offered this by your GP, feel free to ask.

If you're concerned you have a family history of or early risk factors for: bowel, ovarian or breast cancers; diabetes; thyroid problems or osteoporosis, talk to your GP about whether you need early screening or monitoring.

Follicle-stimulating hormone test

While there's no medical need to check if you're perimenopausal or close to menopause itself, for some women it can be useful to know. For instance, if they're experiencing distressing problems with their periods, and want to know if it's the perimenopause or there's another cause. Or if they're still trying for a baby and want to know how viable that is. The way to do this is to check your levels of follicle-stimulating hormone (FSH). FSH is the main hormone that stimulates immature eggs (follicles) in your ovaries to mature into eggs that can be fertilized. As we age, the ovaries become resistant to the effect of FSH so more of it is produced. If your FSH levels are consistently above a certain level, it's likely to be due to the perimenopause. The higher they are, the closer to menopause itself you are. You'll probably need two to three tests on separate days to get a proper picture of your status, as hormone levels can fluctuate from day to day.

Home urine tests

These can be bought from a chemist. They're similar to pregnancy tests and involve urinating on a testing stick. The results usually show up as lines that indicate positive or negative results. Your urine first thing in the morning contains the highest level of FSH so this is the best time to perform the test. Avoid drinking a lot of fluids beforehand as this will dilute the urine and may affect results. Be aware that FSH may be somewhat elevated during the first half of your cycle (before ovulation). If you have a positive result, it's sometimes worth re-testing in case this elevation in FSH is due to your normal menstrual cycle. If you do a home test, it's worth getting your GP to confirm your results.

Tests at your GP's surgery

These usually involve taking a blood sample. The doctor may also test your blood for oestrogen and luteinizing hormone (LH) levels.

Perimenopause energy synchronization

This part of a woman's life cycle is the five to ten years prior to the menopause when her period stops. In other words, this is pre-menopause. For many women this stage of life is full on. Your career might be in full swing. You are probably working your butt off. If it's not about your job and career, you may have even greater stress dealing with financial issues or money shortages. Then there are the personal and home requirements, too. Many of you probably have kids who are still dependent on you. And some will have parents who are also in need. It's a very busy, often stressful and intensive time. This is when illness, sickness and disease has the best chance of breaking in. Your emotions and mental state may suffer as well. You may feel overwhelmed.

However, if you are fully aware of the challenges during this stage and in touch with who you really are, then you will not only get through but fly. This is an opportunity to turn it all around. You can literally and figuratively flip a switch from one direction to the other, from darkness into light.

Because all of the energy centres are in transition at this stage, it is helpful to address all the energy regions throughout the body in a fully integrated manner.

Gillian's diet tips

Eat green vegetables every day, such as spinach, kale, cavolo nero, pak choi, broccoli, lettuce, rocket and Brussels sprouts, to name a few.

Eat foods high in essential fatty acids, including fish, raw shelled hemp seeds, pumpkin seeds, linseeds, sunflower seeds, Brazil nuts, almonds, cashews. Be sure to also eat brown rice, millet and quinoa.

- Protein is important. Sources include tofu, miso, fish, lentils and beans.

- Include ginger, turmeric, coriander, cumin, saffron, fennel and caraway seeds to support your digestion.

Supplement and herb tips

Always consult your medical doctor before embarking on a course of supplements and check with a herbalist for the correct dosage of herbs.

- Include herbs such as basil, parsley, coriander, thyme, sage and chervil. Check out motherwort (especially useful for palpitations or high blood pressure) and hawthorn (for problems associated with the heart and circulation).

- Drink nettle, dandelion and sage tea for its nourishing effects.

'This is the opportunity to turn it all around.'

General lifestyle tips

- Chew your food really well and do relax when you eat. Take a few relaxing breaths before you eat and give thanks for your food.

- Stay well hydrated with lots of water, herbs and vegetable juices.

- Exercise: any moderate regular exercise is essential, including dance, walking, stretching and especially swimming, t'ai chi, chi gung and yoga.

- Also make sure you build some weight-bearing exercise into your routine to help strengthen your bones.

- Follow your heart. Take time to think about what you really want to do with your life. Tune into the little voice inside that knows what is right for you. Thinking about what you enjoyed doing most as a child is often the key.

- Sing! Join a local choir or just have a good sing-along in the bath, shower, car – wherever!

- Make sure you incorporate some weight-bearing exercises into your daily life.

- Spend time every day to do the full-body energy synchronization overleaf.

Full body energy synchronization

1. Lie down in a comfortable position (on a mat or bed) in a quiet room and close your eyes. Place your arms to the side with palms facing up. You can also sit in a chair with feet firmly on the ground if more comfortable. Or sit on the floor with your legs crossed. Choose what feels right for you.

2. Listen to your breathing. Simply imagine that you can see your breath slowly coming into your whole body, filling your feet and legs, tummy, chest, back, arms, neck, head; and then imagine you see the breath slowly being exhaled from your body. Watch the inhalations and exhalations for about a minute. You are visualizing and observing your breath.

3. If any feelings of heavy emotions come up, such as anger, sadness, grief, upset, guilt, rage, confusion, bewilderment, disappointment, frustration or anything else, just stay with it for a minute or so. Notice it, and acknowledge it without fear. Know that it is fine and part of healing to take note of feelings. Now imagine that these heavy, low-vibration emotions have some kind of form and say to it that it's fine for it to leave. Visualize it leaving your body and going out of the nearest window into the sky.

4. Continue to listen to the breath and now imagine the light of a white ball slowly swirling around the base of the spine.

5. Then imagine the white ball slowly swirling in the region just above the base. This is the area just above the pubic bone and just below the navel. Continue to listen to your breath.

6 Now visualize the white ball slowly swirling in the tummy region.

7 Then move your attention up to the area of the chest or heart and imagine the swirling ball of white here.

8 Now go to your throat region and imagine the swirling ball of bright white here.

9 Now find the area just above your nose, between your eyes, slightly above the brow. Visualize the swirling ball of white.

10 Finally, bring your attention to the area at the top of your head, sometimes called the 'crown chakra'. Imagine the swirling ball of strong white coming into your head from above and filling your whole body. Lie with it and listen to your breath.

You need not spend more than about thirty seconds on each of the energy regions of your body. So this practice can be done in less than ten minutes. When you have completed it, say out loud or quietly to yourself:

'My energy is free flowing and balanced within myself and connected fully with the Universal Energy.'

Then visualize beautiful rays of white light coming into your whole body from above.

We are a micro-replication of the macro-picture. Just as we have lay-lines or energy centres throughout our own body, so too does the Earth and the Infinite Universe. As you are finishing this practice, ask that your body's energy centres and lay-lines connect fully with the lay-lines and energy strands of the Earth. Visualize energy centres straddling the globe. Now ask that your own energy centres connect with the lay-lines and energy strands of the Infinite Universe. You need not do anything, just ask and be with it.

Perimenopause – conditions

Dry skin and wrinkles

Decreased oestrogen production as the menopause approaches often results in dry, sometimes itchy skin – on the body as well as the face. Plus, as we age, the outer layer of the skin becomes thinner, loses elasticity and is less able to retain moisture. Add to this the fact that your sebaceous glands produce less sebum, collagen is reduced and skin cells divide more slowly (so repair and healing takes longer) and it's easy to see why many forty-something women start spending a fortune on rich, moisturizing anti-wrinkle creams!

Like other skin problems such as acne, how dry or lined your complexion becomes has a lot to do with genetics. Lifestyle is also a major factor – free-radical damage caused by past sun exposure, smoking or pollution, as well as a poor diet, all contribute hugely to how your skin looks and feels. The earlier you start to take responsibility for your health, the better.

What you can do

While a few wrinkles give the face character, no one wants to age before their time. And dry skin can be uncomfortable and dull. There may not be much we can do about genetics, former habits or the simple passing of time. But we certainly can alter our habits *now* to help balance hormones, nourish and hydrate skin, and prevent further damage.

If you want to retain your looks it's vital to stop smoking and avoid exposure to second-hand smoke. Smokers' skin is parched, wrinkled, grey and lifeless with the skin smelling foul, too. And while I'm always reminding you to get out into natural sunlight every day to top up your vitamin D stores, you don't need more than twenty minutes' exposure at the beginning or end of a day. The rest of the time, wear facial sun block and shades. Again, I can spot a sun worshipper at fifty paces – they have thick, dry, leathery skin and age spots.

Gillian's diet and supplement tips

To reduce the effects of free-radical damage which ages skin, eat a diet high in antioxidants such as vitamins A, C, E, zinc and selenium. You'll find them in abundance in the following skin-friendly foods:

- **CARROTS** Rich in beta-carotene which is converted into vitamin A in the body. Beta-carotene is also found in spinach, squash, watercress, pumpkins and apricots.

- **STRAWBERRIES** A great source of vitamin C needed for collagen production and healing. Also found in other berries, grapefruit, lemons, kiwi fruit, tomatoes and bell peppers.

- **ALMONDS** Rich in vitamin E needed for healing and protection. Other sources include sesame seeds, olive oil, walnuts and avocados.

- **PUMPKIN SEEDS** An excellent source of zinc, for skin repair and healing. Other sources of zinc include fish, whole grains and lentils.

- **BRAZIL NUTS** Just two to three will provide your recommended daily amount of selenium.

- **SHELLED HEMP SEEDS** A good source of essential fatty acids (EFAs), needed to keep skin moist. EFAs are also found in oily fish, flaxseeds, pumpkin seeds, avocados and walnuts.

Water is vital for skin health as dehydrated skin is always going to be less than healthy. Drink two litres a day of water (including herbal teas). Avoid alcohol, coffee, fizzy drinks, sugar, fried foods, refined foods and processed or heated fats. These may all have detrimental effects on skin health and appearance.

Supplement and herb tips

Always consult your medical doctor before embarking on a course of supplements and check with a herbalist for the correct dosage of herbs.

Take a daily fish oil or flaxseed oil supplement for the skin-hydrating essential fatty acids it provides.

Evening primrose or borage oil supplements, also rich in essential fats, may help, too.

Diabetes

Having diabetes basically means your body is unable to regulate its blood-sugar levels properly. Carbohydrates or starchy foods are broken down by the body and enter your bloodstream as glucose. If you're healthy, your pancreas produces the hormone insulin, which helps to transport glucose from the bloodstream into your cells, where it's used as energy. If you have diabetes, however, the pancreas does not produce sufficient insulin or the cells become resistant to insulin or a bit of both so the glucose doesn't make it to your cells. If left untreated, raised glucose levels in the blood can damage surrounding tissues, leading to complications such as eye, nerve and kidney problems as well as heart disease.

Symptoms of diabetes to look out for include:

- Increased thirst
- Frequent urination
- Tiredness and fatigue
- Weight loss
- Blurred vision
- Slow wound healing and tendency to infections
- Genital itching and itchy skin generally
  Note: In type 2 diabetes there may be no symptoms.

There are two main types of diabetes: type 1 and type 2. In type 1, the body can't make insulin so sufferers have to monitor their blood glucose levels and inject with insulin as well as following a special diet. This type normally develops in childhood or young adulthood.

By far the most common form, however, is type 2. Of the 2.6 million people in the UK diagnosed with diabetes (and the more than half a million it's believed are yet to be diagnosed), between 85 and 95 per cent have type 2.

In type 2 diabetes, the pancreas continues to produce insulin, but either it does not make enough or the body is unable to use it efficiently. Although a few people still need insulin injections, most can make do with tablets that help their body to make better use of the insulin, alongside a carefully planned dietary and exercise regime. Some people with type 2 diabetes can manage the condition purely through diet and exercise without the need for medications.

Type 2 is also known as non-insulin-dependent or adult-onset diabetes and occurs mostly in adults over forty. Well, that is, it *used* to. Worryingly, it's being seen more and more in younger people, and it goes hand-in-hand with the growing obesity trend in the West. Over 80 per cent of people diagnosed with type 2 diabetes are overweight.

Other causes or risk factors include:

- Genetic predisposition
- History of severe mental health problems
- History of gestational diabetes
- A sedentary lifestyle
- Being black or Asian and over twenty-five
- Metabolic syndrome
- Being overweight
- High blood pressure
- Raised tryglycerides
- Previous heart attack or a stroke
- Polycystic ovarian syndrome (PCOS)
- Impaired glucose tolerance
- Ageing

Changes in oestrogen and progesterone levels during the perimenopause can also affect how your cells respond to insulin, meaning fluctuations in blood sugar become more likely and your risk of developing diabetes increases. (The weight gain, particularly abdominal, that often occurs in your forties can increase your risk as it indicates that your cells are becoming resistant to insulin.)

If you are already diabetic, the perimenopause may cause complications and mean you need to watch your medication dosage. It's easy to mistake perimenopausal symptoms such as dizziness, fluctuating body temperature, irritability and difficulty concentrating for blood-sugar problems – so always check your levels before medicating.

What you can do

If you have been diagnosed with diabetes, this advice will help you to keep your blood-glucose levels under control, maintain energy and lose weight. If you may be at risk, it will help to prevent it.

However, if you have type 1 diabetes, or you are taking insulin or oral medication for type 2, please check with your medical doctor before following any of these recommendations.

Gillian's diet tips

Never skip meals – you need to eat regularly throughout the day to keep your blood-sugar levels stable. So eat little and often – aim for six meals a day: breakfast, snack, lunch, snack, dinner, snack. Eat until you're satisfied. In the evening, make sure your meals are small.

Choose complex, whole grain carbohydrates rather than simple (refined) ones. So that means brown rice instead of white, wholemeal bread instead of white bread, and wholemeal pasta instead of regular. Refined carbohydrates have had their fibre and nutrients (the brown bits!) removed, and act in a similar way to refined sugar when eaten, raising your blood sugar quickly.

Fresh, raw and steamed vegetables are low in calories and high in essential vitamins, minerals and phytonutrients, so eat plenty. Just be mindful that some veggies, such as white potatoes, parsnips, beetroot and carrots, are high in naturally occurring sugars. So always eat these alongside protein foods, such as beans or lentils, to avoid a sugar rush. Green vegetables and fresh salads are great options.

- Fibre-rich foods help to slow the release of glucose into the bloodstream as well as to reduce high cholesterol, common in diabetics. They'll also help to keep your weight down by making you feel fuller for longer. High-fibre foods include brown rice, oats, rye bread, beans, lentils and flaxseeds.

- Oats are particularly recommended as they contain a fibre called beta-glucan which can help with blood-sugar control.

- Choose protein sources that are low in saturated fat, such as fish, white meat, tofu, nuts, seeds, quinoa, amaranth, beans, lentils and whole grains. Protein slows the digestion of carbohydrates and the rate at which they enter the blood.

- Soya beans are another excellent source of protein that also provide phyto-oestrogens, isoflavones and saponins to balance blood sugar. Soya products to add to your diet are: tofu, tempeh, soya yoghurt, miso, natto and tamari soy sauce.

- Essential fatty acids may help to improve glucose tolerance and reduce high triglyceride and cholesterol levels, so include lots of oily fish, flaxseed oil, dark leafy green vegetables, seeds and nuts in your diet.

- Monounsaturated fats have also been found to improve glucose tolerance in those with diabetes. Good sources include olive oil, olives, avocados and nuts.

- Add garlic (preferably raw) to meals as it can help to lower cholesterol and triglyceride levels in the blood.

- Stay well hydrated by drinking at least eight glasses of water daily.

- Needless to say you need to avoid sugar and all foods that contain sugar, like biscuits and cakes. If you want something sweet, make fresh fruits your friends. Blackberries, blueberries, raspberries, cherries and grapefruit are the best choices as they are not too high in fruit sugars. But make sure you eat a non-fruit food afterwards to help to stabilize the glucose release. Do not eat fruits at night.

- Always check the ingredients on the label as sugar is 'hidden' in a surprising number of products, even savoury ones. It comes in many guises, including sucrose, dextrose, glucose, maltose, lactose, corn syrup, golden syrup and treacle to name a few. The best way to avoid them is to steer clear of processed foods in favour of fresh ingredients and home cooking.

- Beware of label claims like 'unsweetened' or 'no added sugar', too. Such foods may still contain ingredients that are high in naturally occurring sugars (like dried fruit or fruit juice concentrates), or unhealthy artificial sweeteners that have been found to interfere with appetite control.

- Saturated and trans fats increase the risk of developing the complications of type 2 diabetes. So avoid fried foods, red meat, processed meats, full-fat dairy products, fast food, most ready meals, hard margarines and products like pastries, pies, cakes and biscuits.

- Alcohol is basically sugar. I have noticed that diabetics often crave alcohol. And they go ahead and indulge in it. This is not a good idea, as you know. If you must have a drink, eat first. But abstaining is always the better option.

- Use herbs and spices to flavour your food instead of salt.

- Cinnamon has excellent blood-sugar-balancing properties and can help to keep levels stable between meals. Add it to porridge or muesli.

Supplement and herb tips

Always consult your medical doctor before taking supplements and check with a herbalist before taking herbs. There is no need to take all of these suggestions at the same time.

- Take a daily vitamin B complex to improve glucose metabolism and energy production.

- An antioxidant formula containing vitamins A, C and E may help to protect against diabetic retinopathy (damage to the retina of the eye).

- Chromium improves blood-glucose levels in type 2 diabetes by increasing insulin sensitivity.

- Magnesium improves insulin blood-sugar control in type 2 diabetes as well as being needed for energy production.

- Many people with type 2 diabetes are found to be zinc deficient, so take a supplement.

- The vitamin-like compound alpha lipoic acid (ALA) is an antioxidant and improves glucose uptake in type 2 diabetes. It may also reduce diabetic nerve damage and reduce pain.

- Co-enzyme Q10 may help to improve the function of insulin-producing cells in the pancreas.

- Glucomannan fibre (from the konjac plant) can help to stabilize blood-sugar levels. Take it twenty minutes before meals with a large glass of water.

- Ispaghula husks and seeds (Psyllium or plantago) provide a mucilaginous fibre that can help to control blood-sugar levels, reduce cholesterol and give a feeling of fullness that can aid weight loss. They must be taken with plenty of water.

Aloe vera juice, bitter melon, cinnamon, gymnema and mistletoe may all help to lower high blood-glucose levels in people with type 2 diabetes.

General lifestyle tips

Exercise helps with blood-sugar management and weight control. Good forms include walking, power walking, swimming, jogging and yoga. Aim for half an hour of moderate-intensity exercise, at least five times a week (check with your GP before starting a high-intensity exercise programme).

Always eat something light before exercising, such as a few oatcakes, so your blood sugar doesn't drop too low. Afterwards, rehydrate with water and a snack and don't wait too long until your next meal.

Excess abdominal fat makes the body less sensitive to insulin so you need to think about reducing your waistline, using the food and exercise tips described here. Don't try to lose weight quickly – a gradual loss of one to two pounds a week is best. If you follow my recommendations you will lose the weight you need to in a balanced and lasting manner.

Hit the sack. People who get fewer than six hours' sleep per night are less sensitive to insulin than those who get eight hours.

Get outside in daylight every day. Vitamin D, formed by the action of sunlight on bare skin, helps to improve the cells' response to insulin. Supplementary vitamin D may be needed during the winter months.

Fibroids

Fibroids are non-malignant growths of muscle tissue on the internal or external wall of your uterus. They can vary in size from a pea to a melon. They are common in women in their thirties and especially in those in their forties – it's thought over 60 per cent of women over forty-five have them (although only half with symptoms). They usually shrink after the menopause. If you *do* have symptoms, they can include:

- Heavy and/or frequent periods, sometimes with blood clots
- Pain during sexual intercourse
- Frequent urination or constipation
- Anaemia and fatigue caused by heavy bleeding
- Abdominal swelling
- Feeling of fullness in the lower stomach
- Lower back pain
- Infertility

Fibroids are thought to be related to oestrogen levels. The contraceptive pill may increase fibroids due to its oestrogen content. They may also grow during pregnancy, when hormone levels are high.

Liver overload and bowel congestion can be underlying factors. This is due to the liver's role in breaking down and eliminating old hormones via the bowel.

As well as age, other factors thought to increase risk are:

- Genetic predisposition
- Early onset of periods
- Ethnic origin – they are more common in women of black African descent
- Being overweight

- Eating a diet high in red meat
- Eating a diet low in green vegetables

What you can do

If you suffer from any of the symptoms above, always consult your GP. He or she may press around your lower abdomen for lumps on your uterus, do a vaginal examination and/or refer you for an ultrasound or MRI scan.

If symptoms are debilitating, low-dose birth-control pills may be recommended. Sometimes an intrauterine system (IUS) containing a small amount of progesterone can help to control heavy bleeding. In other cases drugs to reduce gonadotrophin are recommended – these have the effect of reducing oestrogen. They may have side effects similar to menopausal symptoms but generally reduce heavy bleeding. Once treatment is stopped fibroids may grow back. Sometimes surgery is recommended to remove the fibroids and, rarely, a hysterectomy (to remove your womb).

None of these approaches, however, addresses the underlying imbalances that may be causing the fibroids to grow. My main aim, with a holistic approach, is to balance the female hormones and improve detoxification and elimination naturally. Liver support is essential. The following advice will help to alleviate existing or suspected fibroids, or reduce your risk of getting them.

Gillian's diet tips

Eat a diet high in fibre to aid removal of old hormones. Fruit, vegetables, whole grains, pulses and flaxseeds are all useful.

Include essential fats daily for their anti-inflammatory and hormone balancing effects – that means oily fish, hemp seeds, flaxseeds, pumpkin seeds, sunflower seeds or the cold pressed oils of these seeds.

- Drink nettle tea to replace lost minerals if bleeding is heavy.

- Eat green vegetables every day – these are high in magnesium and B vitamins needed for hormone balance and to reduce pain and cramping. They are also cleansing for your liver and bowel.

- Fill up on foods rich in iron and vitamin C. Iron levels may be low if heavy bleeding is a symptom – find it in kale, molasses, fish, poultry, almonds, figs, watercress, broccoli, prunes and lentils. Vitamin C aids the absorption of iron, so eat plenty of vitamin C-rich fruit and vegetables.

- Use olive oil for its high vitamin E content. Vitamin E is useful for reducing cramps and PMS symptoms which may be exacerbated by fibroids. Vitamin E is also found in olives, avocados and wheatgerm.

- Sea vegetables are useful for breaking down growths such as fibroids. Try kelp, nori, dulse, kombu and arame. Kelp and nori are easy to use as they can be sprinkled onto soups and salads. Use just a small amount at a time as they are very concentrated foods.

- Regular one or two-day detoxes may help to shrink fibroids as they give the liver a chance to clear out toxins and hormones.

- Avoid coffee, tea, chocolate, dairy products, and non-organic meat and eggs, as they may all disrupt hormone levels and challenge your liver.

Supplement and herb tips

Always consult your medical doctor before taking supplements and check with a herbalist for the correct dosage of herbs. There is no need to take all of these suggestions at the same time.

- Magnesium is vital for female hormone balance.

- Take B vitamins. Vitamin B6 in particular works well with magnesium to rebalance female hormones.

- Take agnus castus every morning to help balance oestrogen and progesterone.

- Take milk thistle tincture and drink dandelion root coffee – both may support your liver.

- Evening primrose oil may help to balance female hormones and can have an anti-inflammatory effect.

General lifestyle tips

- Lose weight if you need to. More fat generally means more oestrogen.

- Improve circulation to the area: hot and cold showers, dry skin brushing, massage and exercise can all aid circulation and remove congestion.

Hot flushes and night sweats

Hot flushes during the day and sweating at night are two of the best known symptoms of the perimenopause. It's thought hormone changes affect the body's vasodilation system (so blood vessels can suddenly dilate, increasing blood flow and heat throughout the body). Not all women will experience them and about 20 per cent of women won't notice them at all. If you have a sudden menopause (if you have surgery to remove your ovaries, for example, or undergo chemotherapy or radiotherapy), symptoms can be more severe.

What you can do
Your GP may suggest hormone replacement therapy (HRT) to reduce symptoms. I would urge you to try these alternative approaches first. (For more on HRT, see page 214.)

Gillian's diet tips

> Sip cool water with lemon.

> Cut out known triggers like spicy foods.

> Add tofu, tempeh and miso to your diet.

> Eat an abundance of fruit and veg.

> Drink sage tea twice a day. If night sweats are a problem, have a cup an hour before bed. Sage is great for reducing sweating.

> Avoid caffeine, alcohol, sugar and refined carbohydrates.

> Stay hydrated by drinking plenty of water – very important if you're losing more water than usual through sweat.

Moroccan chickpea salad

SERVES 2 AS A MAIN COURSE OR 4 AS A SIDE DISH

Can be made in advance and will keep well for
2–3 days covered in the fridge

100g brown rice
2 tbsp olive oil
2 tbsp water
1 medium onion, sliced
1 leek, sliced
1 clove garlic, crushed
1 tsp ground cumin
$\frac{1}{2}$ tsp ground coriander
$\frac{1}{2}$ tsp cinnamon
400g tin chickpeas drained and rinsed in cold water
50g frozen peas
Juice of 1 lemon
2 tbsp freshly chopped coriander
50g baby spinach leaves

1 Place the rice in a medium-sized pan of cold water, bring to the boil, cover and allow to simmer for 20–25 minutes or until tender.

2 Meanwhile, heat the oil and water in a medium-sized frying pan, add the onion and leek and cook gently for 8 minutes. Stir in the garlic and spices, cook for 2 minutes stirring regularly. Remove from the heat and allow to cool.

3 Drain the cooked rice and rinse in cold water.

4 Transfer the rice to a large bowl and add the spiced onion mixture, chickpeas, peas, lemon juice and coriander.

Arrange the spinach leaves on a serving plate and top with the salad.

Sage soup

There's a decent amount of soup here and that's because I want you to freeze some of it, so you have it on hand when you need it. Sage is well-renowned for its effect in reducing excess sweat common with hot flushes.

2 red onions, chopped
3 cloves garlic, peeled and chopped
4 carrots, peeled and chopped
1 head broccoli, florets only
1 white cabbage, shredded
6 new potatoes, halved
3 litres boiling water plus 5 tsp miso powder
1 bag or large handful fresh sage
1 bag or large handful fresh parsley plus extra to garnish

1 Place all the ingredients except the sage and parsley in a large pan, bring to the boil, cover and simmer for 20–30 minutes. Toss the parsley and sage in at the end. Do not cook the sage and parsley.

2 Remove from the heat and blend until smooth.

3 Spoon into large warm bowls and sprinkle with extra parsley.

Supplement and herb tips

Always consult your medical doctor before taking supplements and check with a herbalist for the correct dosage of herbs.

- Citrus bioflavonoids with vitamin C may be helpful.

- Red clover tea or tincture can also be helpful for its phyto-oestrogenic effects.

- Cool down from night sweats by making an infusion of sage, spearmint and lavender. Steep the leaves together for ten minutes, strain and drink.

- Other useful herbs for flushes and sweats include black cohosh, motherwort, red clover and hops. Visit a herbalist to get a prescription specifically for you. Do it!

General lifestyle tips

- Wear lots of thin layers of clothing, in natural fibres, so you can remove or add layers to adjust your temperature.

- Shower in water that's at room temperature.

- Keep your bedroom cool and have a fan near your bed at night.

- Have bed linen and nightclothes made from natural fibres.

- Keep a spritz bottle with you to cool down during a flush. Add the herb sage to this.

- Stress makes symptoms worse, so learn relaxation techniques such as t'ai chi, yoga, meditation or simply deep breathing.

- Take regular exercise.

Joint pain

Some women find they experience general aches and pains in their joints during perimenopause, and may worry it's an injury, virus or early-onset arthritis. Although these shouldn't be discounted, joint pain is more likely to be caused by hormones. Oestrogen and progesterone increase the flexibility and suppleness of the joints, so as they decline over the decade, aches and pains may result.

What you can do

Whatever the cause of joint pain, carrying excess weight will make it worse so try to keep your weight in check with a healthy diet and regular exercise.

Gillian's diet and supplement tips

Always consult your medical doctor before taking supplements and check with a herbalist for the correct dosage of herbs.

- Essential fats are a joint-health must, specifically omega-3 polyunsaturated fatty acids, thanks to their anti-inflammatory and lubricating properties. Increase your intake of oily fish, nuts and seeds or cold-pressed oils used in salad dressings. Consider a fish-oil or flaxseed supplement, too.

- Eat a wide range of fruit and vegetables, in every colour, to ensure you get the full range of antioxidants – important to reduce inflammation and repair body tissues.

- Glucosamine and chondroitin supplements may help, too. Seek advice on the correct dosage.

Drink water to keep your joints hydrated. Herbal teas are also useful, particularly nettle and dandelion which supply nutrients and reduce water retention which can put pressure on the joints.

Saturated fats, processed fats and fatty meats are pro-inflammatory and should be avoided. This means saying no to high-fat dairy products, most sausages, burgers and bacon, margarines and similar products, fried foods and processed foods such as crisps.

Although you probably don't have arthritis, do read up on it and follow the preventative advice on page 393.

Metabolic syndrome

This name is given to a group of risk factors which are increasingly found together in the West. The symptoms all relate to cardiovascular health, blood-sugar control and weight. Being in a pro-inflammatory state is also part of the picture. A diagnosis of metabolic syndrome is made if a patient exhibits abdominal obesity or excess weight around the middle – weight carried in this part of the body puts you at greater risk of many degenerative diseases as compared to weight carried on the hips or thighs. A waist measurement of more than 80cm (31in) in women and 94cm (36in) in men indicates central obesity. Plus any two of the following:

- High blood pressure – above 130/85 or receiving treatment to lower blood pressure.

- High fasting blood-glucose levels of more than 5.6mmol/l or receiving treatment for high blood sugar.

- High triglycerides – triglycerides are a type of fat found in the blood. Levels tend to increase when calories are consumed but not used up for energy.

- Decreased HDL cholesterol – HDL cholesterol is a beneficial type of cholesterol that is associated with a reduced risk of cardiovascular disease.

Women with metabolic syndrome are at increased risk of heart attacks, strokes, atherosclerosis, diabetes and polycystic ovaries. About 80 per cent of people with type 2 diabetes are thought to have metabolic syndrome.

The likelihood of metabolic syndrome increases dramatically in women in the six years before and after the menopause due to the reduction in oestrogen and progesterone levels and the relative increase in testosterone at this time. These hormonal changes mean weight is more likely to be gained around the middle, rather than on the hips, thighs and breasts as may be the case in younger women. Abdominal weight gain is very much a symptom of metabolic syndrome and all its associated diseases.

Other risk factors include:

- A family history of type 2 diabetes
- High blood pressure
- High blood triglycerides
- Polycystic ovaries
- A sedentary lifestyle
- Being overweight
- Having a waist measurement of 80cm (31in) or more in women and 94cm (36in) in men
- Low birth weight
- Insulin resistance – this is one of the major features of metabolic syndrome

- High testosterone levels in women
- Diet high in refined carbohydrates, sugar and refined vegetable oils and low in omega-3 fats and fresh fruit and vegetables

One of the most common causes of metabolic syndrome is a diet high in sugar, refined carbohydrates and alcohol – foods that break down into glucose once digested. This glucose enters the bloodstream causing a rapid and dramatic rise in blood-sugar levels. Now because your body can't survive if blood-sugar levels are constantly high, insulin is secreted by the pancreas in order to transport glucose into your cells. There it's either stored for later use as energy or converted to fat for long-term storage.

Insulin is a storage hormone that likes to store glucose rather than release it for energy. Therefore, the more insulin you produce the more likely you are to convert glucose to fat. And you can end up storing it as fat, particularly around the middle of the body.

Diets high in sugar, refined carbohydrates and alcohol mean insulin is constantly being called upon to carry the glucose into the cells. This can lead to the cells becoming 'deaf' to insulin, or 'insulin resistant' as they get so used to it being present. More and more is secreted until the cells let the glucose enter. As, by now, insulin levels are higher than they should be, more glucose is stored as fat and less is available for energy. This leads to the deposition of fat around the middle of the body, hence the characteristic apple shape that's become more common in women as they age.

What you can do

The key for prevention and treatment is to lose weight. You also need to follow sensible heart-health advice.

Gillian's diet tips

Eating regularly spaced small meals and snacks is a *must*. Have six small meals and snacks a day rather than the traditional three (you don't need to eat more over the day, you just space out the portions). Large meals always provoke a rise in blood glucose and insulin levels.

Protein slows the breakdown of carbohydrates into glucose so include some at every meal. Good combinations include chicken or fish with vegetables (not potatoes) or lentils, beans, soya, nuts or seeds with whole grains such as brown rice, oats, quinoa, millet, buckwheat and amaranth.

Make sure all your meals and snacks contain fibre from whole grains, nuts, seeds, fruit, vegetables, beans or pulses. Fibre helps to keep insulin levels low and blood sugar stable. Oats are particularly recommended as they contain a fibre called beta-glucans which can help with blood-sugar control after meals – plus it reduces cholesterol.

Omega-3 essential fatty acids found in oily fish have protective and anti-inflammatory effects on the cardiovascular system and can improve cellular response to insulin. Vegetarian sources of omega-3s include flaxseeds, hemp seeds, pumpkin seeds, walnuts and avocados (and their cold-pressed oils).

Eat at least five portions of fruit and vegetables a day. Eight servings is even better. A high consumption of fruit and vegetables is associated with reduced blood pressure, improved cholesterol levels, reduced weight and better health overall.

- It is important to avoid refined vegetable oils and to choose cold-pressed fats instead. Particularly beneficial are the mono-unsaturated fats found in olive oil, olives, avocados and nuts, such as almonds.

- Garlic has protective effects on the cardiovascular system. Use it raw and in cooking.

- Eat potassium-rich foods such as apricots, avocados, prunes, figs, green vegetables, peas, lentils and beans. Potassium is needed for cardiovascular health and to balance sodium which, if unchecked, can lead to high blood pressure.

- You need to avoid all foods that break down into glucose rapidly as they'll only increase insulin levels and the conversion of glucose to fat. Foods to avoid include sugar, soft drinks, alcohol, biscuits, cakes, pastries, chocolate, sweets, white pasta, white rice, white bread, white flour products, crisps and potatoes.

- A high salt intake raises blood pressure, one of the risk factors for metabolic syndrome, so no adding salt to cooking or foods, and avoid high-salt products.

- Avoid stimulants such as tea, coffee, colas and cigarettes. These all contain nicotine or caffeine which indirectly raises blood-sugar levels and therefore insulin.

Supplement and herb tips

Always consult your medical doctor before taking supplements and check with a herbalist for the correct dosage of herbs. There is no need to take all of these suggestions at the same time.

- A daily chromium picolinate supplement may help. Chromium has anti-diabetic, anti-obesity, blood-pressure-lowering and cholesterol-lowering properties.

- Supplementing with alpha lipoic acid (ALA) may help to improve glucose uptake by muscle cells, meaning less glucose is stored as fat. Alpha lipoic acid (not to be confused with alpha linolenic acid) is a fatty acid found in every cell of the body. One of its main roles is in aiding the conversion of glucose to energy, thus helping with blood-sugar control. It also functions as an antioxidant and helps to maintain levels of other antioxidants such as vitamin C and glutathione in the body. Alpha lipoic acid can be made in the body as well as being found in small amounts in some foods such as spinach, chard, Brewer's yeast, broccoli, peas and rice bran.

- Co-enzyme Q10 may improve the function of insulin-producing cells in the pancreas.

- The B vitamins play a key role in blood-sugar control, energy production and cardiovascular health so I'd recommend a B-complex supplement daily.

- Likewise magnesium citrate which is needed for blood-sugar control, energy and cardiovascular health.

- Take glucomannan fibre. Research has shown that glucomannan from the plant konjac can help to reduce the surge in insulin after meals. You can find it in health-food stores in the form of capsules or powder. Drink plenty of water when taking it as it is highly soluble and absorbs many times its own weight in water, meaning it gives a feeling of fullness. Take it on an empty stomach or at least twenty minutes before meals.

General lifestyle tips

> Being overweight puts you at increased risk of all the other factors associated with the syndrome, so losing weight needs to be your priority.

> Not only does regular exercise help you to lose weight, it also improves your cells' response to insulin, normalizes appetite and reduces cravings. It increases levels of 'good' HDL cholesterol, lowers blood pressure and supports heart health.

> Vitamin D is manufactured in the skin in response to sunlight, and it has been shown to improve the cellular response to insulin. Make sure you get outside in daylight with some skin exposed every day and consider a vitamin D supplement during the winter months.

'If you are fully aware of the challenges during this stage and in touch with who you really are, then you will not only get through, but fly.'

Mood swings

Fluctuating hormone levels during perimenopause, as well as psychological issues raised by declining fertility or other life changes, can mean depression, anxiety, irritability, feeling teary and other tricky mind states which all make life difficult from time to time. (For every down there's usually an up, though, so it's not all doom and gloom!)

What you can do

Your blood-sugar levels have a huge effect on mood, so look at and follow the advice on mood swings I give in the section on Puberty (page 74) – it's no less relevant to you now. In addition, the general advice I give on balancing hormones during the perimenopause is vital (see page 217).

Exercise has an incredibly positive effect on mood – all the better if you can do it outside. The action of daylight on the pineal gland helps to control our daily rhythms and moods. I'm a big believer in the balancing, mood-stabilizing effect of acupuncture, too.

If circumstances (divorce, separation, job loss, bereavement) are contributing to your moods, it's worth seeking out a talk therapist. And if low moods continue for more than two weeks consistently or are affecting your ability to live a normal life, see your GP.

Gillian's diet and supplement tips

Always consult your medical doctor before taking supplements and check with a herbalist for the correct dosages before taking herbs.

> While a healthy diet should be low in saturated and trans fats, remember you still need essential fats for the production of hormones and neuro-transmitters in the brain that control mood.

> St John's wort has been shown to be as effective as conventional antidepressant medications, without the side effects, for mild to moderate depression. Consult your medical practitioner before taking it as it can interact badly with some medications, including oral contraceptives and warfarin. It can increase photo-sensitivity so if you take it avoid going outside between 11am and 3pm or your skin may react.

> The herb rhodiola and the vitamin supplement L-theanine are both fast-acting and particularly good for anxiety.

> The herb black cohosh may aid mood control while motherwort may be soothing. The following herbs may be helpful too: ashwaganda, Siberian ginseng, ginkgo biloba or dong quai.

> The spice saffron, used in tiny amounts (just a few strands), can promote emotional stability. Add it at the end of cooking to rice and vegetables.

Palpitations or rapid heartbeat

During the perimenopause, some women report symptoms ranging from a slight 'flutter' of an irregular heartbeat to feeling as if their heart is going to beat right out of their chest. Sometimes the problem occurs alone, at other times it accompanies hot flushes or anxiety attacks. Either way it can be frightening. Lower levels of progesterone relative to oestrogen may be responsible for irregular or rapid heartbeats during the perimenopause. Progesterone tends to have a relaxing effect, so the relative deficiency of progesterone may be at least partly responsible for irregularities in the heart rhythm.

Non-hormonal causes include stress, anxiety, stimulants such as caffeine and nicotine, and nutrient deficiencies.

All palpitations or rapid heartbeats must be reported to your medical doctor.

What you can do

- Reduce sodium and increase potassium. These two nutrients need to be in balance with each other for a healthy heart and cardiovascular system. Avoid processed and packaged foods and increase your consumption of fresh fruit, vegetables, beans and lentils. Even a banana would be a good start.

- Flavour your foods with herbs and mild spices instead of relying on salt.

- Green vegetables are particularly beneficial for their magnesium content.

- To help balance the hormones, phyto-oestrogens from soya, red clover and linseeds may help.

- Essential fats are also important for hormonal balance as well as heart function, so include pumpkin seeds, hemp seeds, sunflower seeds and linseeds every day and oily fish a couple of times a week.

- Keep blood-sugar levels stable as insulin can upset female hormone balance. Eat little and often and avoid sugar and refined carbohydrates.

- Avoid coffee, chocolate and nicotine. These are all stimulants which may raise your heartbeat and trigger palpitations if you're prone. Drink herbal teas, water and vegetable juices instead.

- Learn to manage stress. Yoga, t'ai chi, meditation and breathing exercises are all good daily practices.

- Get your bahookee moving. That means regular, moderate exercise but avoid overdoing it. Walking, swimming, cycling, dancing, rebounding exercises and jogging are all good ways to improve cardiovascular health.

Tiredness and lack of energy

Many women at this stage of life find that they have less energy and feel tired more often than they did in their younger years. However, this is definitely not inevitable. The main causes are blood-sugar imbalances, thyroid problems, insomnia (possibly caused by anxiety, depression or night sweats) and weight gain. And of course you may lack energy because of insufficient exercise. Many women feel tired without any known cause. Some medical doctors think it is because of a fall in testosterone.

What you can do

My general advice for coping with perimenopause (see page 217) should be heeded, and if you suspect you may have a thyroid or blood-sugar problem (see 'Metabolic syndrome', page 261) or are depressed, read up on these conditions, too.

Gillian's diet tips

- Eat little and often to keep blood-sugar levels stable. The sugar in your blood is what provides you with energy for physical and mental activity. So don't skip meals!

- Complex carbohydrates break down slowly into glucose, meaning your energy will stay stable for longer. Good sources include brown rice, oats, quinoa, lentils and beans.

- B vitamins and magnesium are two of the key nutrients needed for energy production in the body. They are found in whole grains, green vegetables, pumpkin seeds, almonds, fish and bananas.

- Avoid sugar and refined carbohydrates. These may provide an initial lift but this is followed by a slump. They zap nutrients and energy and provide empty calories.

- Avoid alcohol, caffeine and cigarettes – these all have a negative effect on blood sugar and stimulate the adrenal glands, which can become exhausted if these substances are taken over a period of years.

Supplement and herb tips

Always consult your medical doctor before taking supplements and check with a herbalist for the correct dosage of herbs. There is no need to take all of these suggestions at the same time.

- Astragalus, Siberian ginseng and rhodiola are all useful for long-term fatigue. You can even drink them as teas.

- Liquorice tea first thing in the morning can help to give a caffeine-free boost. (Liquorice should not be taken if you have, or are at risk of, high blood pressure.)

- Magnesium is needed for the production of energy within the cells. It also has a relaxing effect on the muscles and nerves so is good if tiredness is due to frazzled nerves.

- B vitamins are also needed for the production of energy. Take a B complex every morning to give yourself a lift. Make sure you take this supplement with food, not on an empty stomach.

- Co-enzyme Q10 is needed for energy production. Normally, the body makes its own co-enzyme Q10, but production levels tend to diminish with age.

Energy booster berry and banana smoothie

Combine a banana with a handful of strawberries and a teaspoon of spirulina or another green superfood powder. Bananas supply magnesium and B vitamins needed for energy. Berries supply vitamin C which is often needed when you are tired from burning the candle at both ends.

Sunflower seeds are a nice little pick-me-up, too.

General lifestyle tips

It might be the last thing you feel like if you're exhausted, but make time for exercise. Believe me, it *gives* you energy. Just avoid overdoing it and build up gradually – you don't have to run a marathon! Be sure to eat well after exercise as complex carbohydrates are needed to refuel your energy stores and protein is needed to repair muscle tissue. If you don't replenish your body with nutrients, exercise will leave you feeling tired. It is also important not to exercise within three hours of going to bed as this can interfere with a good night's sleep, meaning you wake up feeling tired.

Get to bed at a reasonable hour and aim for a good seven hours' sleep. Ideally, be in bed before eleven o'clock each night. (Aim for ten o'clock, that way you should make it by half-past ten!) Every hour you can clock before midnight is worth two after.

Learn relaxation techniques. Yoga, t'ai chi and breathing exercises can all improve energy.

Urinary tract infections

Half of all women will experience a urinary tract infection (UTI) during their lifetime and they're fifty times more common in women than men. Although uncomfortable and upsetting, they're not usually harmful – but should always be addressed, as complications can be serious. The most common UTIs that affect the lower part of the urinary system – the urethra and bladder – include urethritis and cystitis. If you've ever had a UTI, you've probably just called it cystitis.

Symptoms include frequent, painful and burning urination (or wanting to urinate but nothing comes out) and cloudy, dark-coloured urine. There may be blood in the urine, an ache or pain in the lower abdomen and a general feeling of being unwell.

UTIs are usually caused by bacterial infection of the urethra, vagina or sometimes the kidneys, with E. coli. This usually lives harmlessly in the bowel but can be transferred to the urethra and up into the bladder. Urinalysis will show a high number of white blood cells and bacteria.

We women are more susceptible than men for anatomical reasons: the female urethra and anus are closer together, and the urethra itself is shorter, so bacteria has less distance to cover before it reaches the bladder.

UTIs are more likely to occur if:

- You don't wipe from front to back after using the loo.

- You're post or perimenopausal. Low oestrogen levels cause loss of tissue elasticity and vaginal dryness and a thinned lining of the urethra and bladder which is more likely to be infected.

- You have frequent, vigorous sex which can lead to an inflamed urethra and make infection more likely (known as honeymoon cystitis).

- You have thrush which causes inflammation of the vagina. This is often a problem in those with recurring cystitis.

- You're diabetic (sugar in the urine encourages bacteria to multiply).

- You use irritating soaps, shower gels, douches, other toiletries or spermicides.

- You are constipated.

Other possible causes of UTIs:

- Some contraceptive devices may increase the risk of infection due to their detrimental effect on the vaginal microflora.

- Dehydration caused by insufficient fluid intake or excess diuretics.

- Substances in the urine that irritate the bladder such as additives, spices, acidic foods (meat, dairy, sugar), coffee, tea, alcohol, some fruit juices, colas and food allergens.

- A compromized immune function.

Interstitial cystitis is characterized by inflammation of the bladder but with no infection present. The epithelial lining of the bladder and urethra is damaged and becomes inflamed. The tight junctions between epithelial cells are damaged causing increased permeability meaning inflammatory substances can migrate to the urine causing pain.

If a UTI continues up past the bladder to the ureter or kidneys, it can be much more serious, so it's important to catch it early. Symptoms of an upper UTI to look out for include feeling systemically unwell, a fever, shakes and shivering, pain on one side, vomiting or diarrhoea.

What you can do

If you have symptoms of an upper UTI you must see your GP immediately or even go to A&E. The infection could be spreading up to your kidneys, putting you at risk of a life-threatening condition, pyelonephritis.

In the case of lower UTIs/cystitis, medical doctors usually prescribe antibiotics. However, this can lead to resistant bacterial strains and a disturbance in the microflora. I believe there's plenty you can do yourself to deal with and prevent UTIs – but do see your GP if there's no improvement after forty-eight hours or your infections keep coming back. If you're peri- or post-menopausal, a low-dose oestrogen cream you apply to the area may help to prevent but not treat the condition. Always see your GP if you're pregnant or diabetic and have symptoms.

Gillian's diet tips

- If you are a regular sufferer of this condition, it's a good idea to keep a food diary to see if anything triggers it or makes things worse.

- It's essential to stay well hydrated all the time as this will help to flush bacteria out of your bladder before it has time to take hold. Drink plenty during an attack, even though it's the last thing you might want to do. The more concentrated your urine is, the more uncomfortable you'll be.

- Drink sugar-free cranberry and/or blueberry juice and add the berries to fruit smoothies. Research shows their active ingredient, hippuric acid, prevents bacteria from sticking to your bladder walls. This is particularly good if you're prone to repeated attacks, as a preventative measure.

- Drink barley water to rejuvenate the kidneys. To make this, simmer ½ cup of pot barley in 5 cups of water. Add a cinnamon stick or grated ginger if you like. Simmer for 20 minutes, cool and strain, and drink throughout the day. You can add a squeeze of lemon for extra flavour and cleansing properties.

- Cinnamon, garlic, onions, oregano, thyme, ginger, fenugreek, chicory and nettles may all reduce infection and inflammation so add them to cooking.

- Eat plenty of fresh fruit and vegetables, nuts and seeds, flax and hemp oils.

- Steer clear of substances that will hang around in your urine and irritate your bladder, such as those found in additives, spices, acidic foods (meat, dairy, sugar, processed foods), caffeine, alcohol, fruit juices and fizzy drinks.

- Other irritating foods may include asparagus, spinach, potatoes, tomatoes, citrus fruits and juices, strawberries, dairy products and chlorinated water.

- Avoid sugar and refined grains as these provide sugar that feeds the bacteria. Use whole grains such as quinoa, brown rice and oats instead.

'If you want to make the most of your forties and fifties, eating healthily and modifying your lifestyle is a must. I'm in no doubt whatsoever that it enables your body to adjust to the changes associated with perimenopause.'

Supplement and herb tips

Always consult your medical doctor before taking a course of supplements and if taking herbs, check with a herbalist for the correct dosage.

- Daily cranberry extract tablets can help if you're prone to repeated bouts.

- Take a daily probiotic supplement for good gut health, strong immunity and to help prevent the overgrowth of the yeast candida. Probiotics, cranberry and mannose have all been shown to be useful in preventing a recurrence of UTIs in the long term.

- Goldenseal and uva ursi can be supplemented for their antibacterial properties. I recommend taking them with nettle and dandelion teas and linseeds.

- Juniper berries, buchu, burdock, cleavers, parsley and shavegrass are helpful, too. Seek the help of a herbalist to create a herbal prescription specifically for you.

- Vitamin C with bioflavonoids to stimulate the immune system and hinder bacterial growth.

- Vitamin E is protective and enhances the immune response.

General lifestyle tips

- Ensure the bowels are moving two to three times a day – see section on constipation (page 174) if this is a problem for you.

- Wipe from front to back after using the loo.

- Get up and pass water as soon as possible after sexual intercourse, to flush away any bacteria that may have entered the urethra.

- Avoid perfumed toiletries and so-called 'feminine hygiene' products such as douches, intimate deodorants and wipes.

- Use natural cotton sanitary products to avoid irritation in the area. Tampons may exacerbate the problem so alternatives are often better.

- Bacteria love warm, moist conditions so wear cotton underwear, go 'commando' at night and avoid tight trousers. Don't sit around in wet swimwear after going to the pool or beach.

- Don't 'hold on' if you need to pee and sit down to do it, never 'hover' over the seat or you won't empty your bladder properly.

- A cup of apple cider vinegar with a few drops of eucalyptus, bergamot, lavender or juniper essential oils makes a soothing bath during an attack.

Vaginal dryness

Declining oestrogen levels due to the perimenopause can lead to changes in the mucous secretions of the vagina meaning many women experience vaginal dryness during and after the menopause. The mucus that normally occurs in the vagina keeps the vaginal walls thick and lubricated. With less oestrogen, the vaginal walls can become thin and dry. At best, this can be itchy and make sex uncomfortable; at worst it can be painful and cause cracks, bleeding and make sex impossible. It may also increase the chance of developing vaginitis and susceptibility to infections.

What you can do

You GP can prescribe a topical oestrogen cream, suppositories or a vaginal ring to remoisturize the area. This is a very low-dose form of local HRT. There are also plenty of topical lubricants and intimate moisturizers you can buy over the counter. As ever, I'd recommend natural alternatives in preference.

Gillian's diet and supplement tips

Always consult your medical doctor before taking a course of supplements and, if taking herbs, check with a herbalist for the correct dosage.

Make sure you get plenty of essential fats in your diet daily: oily fish (mackerel, salmon, sardines, pilchards, herrings and trout), raw shelled hemp seeds, flaxseeds, pumpkin seeds, sunflower seeds, walnuts and avocados are all good sources. Their anti-inflammatory and moisturizing action will help.

- Flaxseeds are particularly helpful as they contain plant oestrogens called lignans that may help to improve oestrogen balance and relieve symptoms such as vaginal dryness. Grind them in a coffee grinder or seed mill and sprinkle a tablespoon or two onto your food each day.

- Take the herb black cohosh in tincture form, twice a day. Other useful herbs may include red clover, liquorice, calendula, American ginseng, false unicorn, motherwort and wild yam.

- Supplement with vitamin E daily. The foods listed above for their essential fat content are also good sources of vitamin E, as is olive oil. You can also apply vitamin E oil topically by piercing open a vitamin-E capsule and massaging the oil into the vagina every night. This helps to heal cracks and reduces dryness.

- Dandelion leaf and oat-straw teas can both be beneficial for their nutritive effects.

- Aloe vera gel can be applied topically to soothe and heal.

- Natural progesterone cream works for some women. It is best to discuss this with your doctor first.

- Avoid washing the area with soap and steer clear of bubble baths and vaginal perfumes or synthetic products.

- Regular sex helps to keep the vaginal wall elastic and maintains a healthy blood supply to the area.

- Evening primrose oil is helpful for improving essential fatty acid balance and female hormone balance.

Q: Dear Gillian,

I'm in my forties and I have the complexion of a teenager. My skin is greasy, covered in spots. I even get spots on my back and sometimes my chest. To add insult to injury, I'm now noticing wrinkles, too! Can I really have acne – at my age? And, if not, why am I so spotty?

Alex, 42

A: Dear Alex,

You'd be amazed how many adults still struggle with spots and greasy skin. Modern life often leads to hormonal imbalances, nutrient deficiencies, poor diet, liver overload and poor elimination via the bowel which may all be contributing to the problem. Stress and pollution also take their toll on skin.

Make sure you're eating a healthy diet. Sugar, refined carbohydrates, processed foods, alcohol, caffeine, dairy products, chocolate and additives can all clog up the skin and need to be eliminated.

Cleansing the liver and bowel is a good way of clearing skin. Eat a diet rich in raw fruit and vegetables – full of nutrients needed for healthy skin and cleansing to the liver and bowel. Whole grains such as brown rice, quinoa, oats and millet are great for improving elimination, so eat these daily. It is also important to stay well hydrated. Drink eight large glasses of water a day. Herbal drinks are also cleansing, especially nettle tea and dandelion coffee.

Give your body a cleansing rest once a month for the next three months and see your skin improve. During a cleanse, eat mainly raw fruit and vegetables and sprouted pulses and seeds and drink vegetable juices and herbal teas.

Zinc and vitamin A are often low in those with acne. Zinc is found in pumpkin seeds, fish, chicken, lentils and flaxseeds. Vitamin A can be made in the body from beta-carotene found in carrots, apricots, squash, pumpkins, watercress and broccoli.

If hormonal imbalances seem likely, talk to your GP about blood tests and a scan for polycystic ovarian syndrome. It may also be that hormonal changes associated with the perimenopause are affecting your skin – just as they may have in your teenage years. The herb agnus castus often helps with acne caused by imbalances in female hormones. If you are on any other medication consult your GP before taking it.

In terms of topical treatments, try making your own face masks to aid skin healing. Mix oatmeal with honey and olive oil or just apply live natural yoghurt or a mashed avocado or papaya. Clay masks that you can buy from health-food stores can also be effective. Dabbing witch hazel onto spots can reduce the infection and speed healing.

It is essential to get some fresh air, daylight and exercise every day. Dry skin brushing is great for getting the lymphatic system moving and can be done before showering.

See the sections on acne (page 60) and PCOS (page 150) for more ideas.

post-menopause and beyond

It's your 'Wisdom Years' – those decades, post-menopause and beyond, in which women in many cultures are revered for the knowledge and experience they have accumulated in life.

This part of your life can be just as happy and healthy as any other if you choose to look after yourself. I have known so many vibrant, energetic, perky friends and relatives, from their fifties to their eighties, who put younger folks to shame!

In this chapter, I'll be covering your health from your post-menopausal years onwards. Why put all these decades together? Because, these days, the boundaries of age are so blurred it simply wouldn't be relevant to divide them. And the advice and precautions I offer apply just as much at fifty-seven as they do at eighty-seven.

Once you have been through the menopause and your periods have ceased (as defined in the previous section), you're described as being post-menopausal. Although your reproductive years are officially at an end, you may continue to experience a few of the hormone-related symptoms (for which the approaches already described will continue to be effective). But these will gradually settle.

For many women the post-menopausal years are wonderful – a time of freedom and joy. You no longer have to contend with your periods, or risk of pregnancy. Your risk of many health problems, such as endometriosis, fibroids or pre-menstrual syndrome (PMS) diminishes or disappears. You feel mature, self-assured, either in a stable relationship or self-confident in your singledom, have a good career and perhaps more 'me time' if you had kids and they have left home. There's a sense of 'getting your life back'. These days, 'active retirement' is the norm.

But, of course, everyone's different, and for others these years may have additional challenges. Having children later in life (or children who stay at home for longer!) means you could well be looking after a family while also working – and perhaps caring for your own elderly parents. You may never have worked so hard in your life! Or there may be some psychological adjustments as you cope with children leaving (Q&A on 'Empty-nest syndrome', page 402) and the ageing process. Some women find they mourn the loss of their fertile years.

Now, you know me well by now, so I'm sure you can guess what's coming next. That's right – whatever your experience of the decades post menopause, you can make them healthier and more joyous with good nutrition and wise lifestyle habits.

I'm not about to kid you that you can halt the ageing

process completely – time passing and the cumulative effects of gravity will have some inevitable effects of wear and tear on your body and appearance. And there's no denying your lack of oestrogen leaves you more susceptible to certain conditions and diseases of ageing. But that's all the more reason why paying attention to your health now will pay huge dividends. Yes, you may have to work harder at exercise if you want to maintain that toned tush! Your diet may need significant adjustments if you want to avoid abdominal weight gain. But it can be done. Be extra aware, not extra worried. Think of those people you know, be they friends, family or celebrities, who seem to defy their age. I'll bet that's not due to the surgeon's knife or a Botox habit, just good, clean living!

So you're not in your first flush of youth any more. So what? It's all about a youthful outlook. The average life expectancy for women in the UK is eighty and rising.

'We're living longer than our mothers and grandmothers and are healthier and happier and more active than ever.'

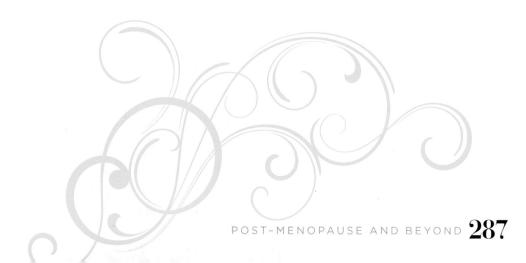

The importance of good nutrition

One of the easiest ways to improve your diet is to adopt a few of my simple rules and suggestions for eating and cooking your food. It's a back-to-basics approach but nonetheless one that will come in really handy, whether you need to make sure you're eating enough, you need to cut down or you need to get into healthier habits. Remember, always make dietary changes gradually, not overnight!

Cook from scratch as much as possible. This means avoiding processed and packaged foods and using whole, natural ingredients. It's the easiest way to maximize your nutrient intake and be sure of what you're putting into your body. When you cook a meal, make extra so that you can heat up the rest the next day. Make stews and casseroles – enough to freeze some in batches for future meals.

Any vegetables can be made into nutritious and delicious soups. For extra protein add lentils and beans (canned is fine as long as contents of the can are simply the beans and water, nothing else. Try chickpeas, aduki, borlotti, butter beans, lentils). Just add water or, for more flavour, vegetable bouillon (look for low-salt varieties), tamari, miso, herbs and mild spices such as ginger. Simmer until the veg is tender then blend with a hand blender or in a liquidizer.

What do you mean you've still got a deep-fat fryer in the cupboard? Bin it – NOW! You can eat vegetables raw and of course there is steaming, baking, poaching and roasting. Here are some easy, nutrient-saving ways to cook:

Steam any vegetable you would normally boil and you'll preserve more of the colour, the crunch and the nutrients. Steaming is faster, too. Use a bamboo or metal steamer that fits inside your normal saucepan.

Vegetables are delicious when roasted, too – the heat breaks down their carbohydrates into sugars, meaning they taste sweeter and are easier to digest. Putting a small amount of olive oil on the vegetables actually helps to seal in the nutrients and enhances their flavour. Most vegetables can be roasted. The only preparation needed is washing, peeling (if necessary) and chopping into large chunks. Try parsnips, carrots, swede, celeriac, beetroots, squash, pumpkin, courgettes, marrows and shitake mushrooms.

Potatoes aren't the only vegetable that can be baked. Sweet potatoes and whole squash (such as butternut or red kuri) can be baked just as you would bake normal white potatoes. Other vegetables can be wrapped in tin foil and baked in the oven – try beetroots and carrots. Yum!

Finally, make time to eat. Sit down, chew thoroughly until your food is liquid and listen to your body. You don't have to eat until you burst. Eat until you feel satisfied.

Top foods for post-menopause and beyond

So now we've tackled how to eat, let's look at my top foods for this stage of your life.

> **VEGETABLES** All types are yours for the eating! Try to take in a range of colours over the week and have something green every day. Dark green leafies are very important for the ladies as they are good sources of bone-building minerals and disease-fighting antioxidants. If you find you don't digest raw veggies well, use some of the cooking methods described above – especially soups. (Cooking breaks down the cellulose walls in vegetables, which can be harder to digest.)

> **FRUIT** Packed full of antioxidants that protect your cells from age-related damage and disease. Soft fruits such as berries, apricots, nectarines and bananas may be easy enough to eat as they are. Others, such as apples or pears, may be better tolerated if cooked gently in a small amount of water with some cinnamon. Smoothies and juices are great if you can make them yourself (some shop-bought varieties are often full of sugar or additives). Soaked dried fruits are also easy and delicious. Look for unsulphured varieties as many contain sulphur dioxide so that they retain their colour. This is not necessary or beneficial.

> **FIBRE** Vital for good digestion and elimination and some of the best sources are whole grains, like brown rice, millet, buckwheat, oats, quinoa, amaranth, barley and rye. Cooking one cup of brown rice to three cups of water is a good ratio to render the grain fibres soft enough and easily digestible. Or experiment with whole grain flakes (in muesli or porridge). Buckwheat, millet and quinoa flakes are especially easy as they can be prepared without cooking.

NUT AND SEED BUTTERS These are available in most supermarkets and health-food shops. They provide a good way of getting the benefits of nuts and seeds if chewing the whole seeds is a problem. Those available include hazelnut, almond, pumpkin seed, sunflower seed, cashew-nut and peanut butters. They can be stirred into porridge or whole grains after cooking or used as spreads on toast and oatcakes to add flavour and essential fats.

SEEDS A great source of essential fats, zinc, magnesium and B vitamins, all of which are needed to maintain health. Include ground pumpkin seeds, sunflower seeds and hemp seeds. They can be sprinkled onto cereal or salads or eaten as snacks. Soaked and ground flaxseeds provide essential anti-inflammatory fats and can help to relieve constipation. Have some in porridge or on cereal, daily.

BEANS AND LENTILS A good source of protein and fibre. Buy canned (without added salt), rinse before use and add to salads, soups, stews, dips and whole grains. Pulses contain phyto-oestrogens which may exert some of the beneficial effects of oestrogen. Chickpeas are a great food to include.

SOYA Contains phyto-oestrogens (see 'Perimenopause', page 229). Soya foods to include are tempeh, tofu, miso, tamari and soya yoghurt. Avoid processed soya products and textured vegetable protein as these do not have the same benefits.

EGGS Provide useful protein, B vitamins, essential fats, zinc and lecithin (which aids fat digestion). Contrary to popular belief ,they do not raise cholesterol, but may be hard to digest for some people, so eat them in moderation. Opt for organic or free-range eggs.

FISH Super-easy to grill, steam, poach or bake. Opt for oily fish such as mackerel and salmon, which provide those essential fatty acids you know I love! They're an excellent protein alternative to red and processed meats and rich in minerals such as zinc, magnesium and selenium. Serve with salad or vegetables for an easy lunch or dinner. Add herbs such as fennel, dill and parsley to aid digestion as well as enhance flavour. While fresh fish is ideal, canned fish is relatively unprocessed, inexpensive and easy to use, too. Tins of mackerel, salmon, sardines and pilchards can make an easy lunch; just drain and add to salads or vegetables.

CALCIUM-RICH FOODS These should be part of your daily diet to help keep your bones healthy. Some folks just can't tolerate dairy but calcium is found in quinoa, broccoli, watercress, kale, Brussels sprouts, almonds, figs, tahini, hazelnuts, chickpeas, oats, haricot beans, fish and sea vegetables as well as natural, unsweetened yoghurts. It's the uptake and digestibility of the calcium that is important. Other nutrients needed for bone health are magnesium (which helps your body to use calcium efficiently) found in green vegetables, seeds and whole grains; vitamin K from green vegetables; and miso and boron from apples, pears and carrots.

SEA VEGETABLES Rich in iodine needed for thyroid function. They are also an excellent source of many other minerals, including calcium, magnesium and potassium.

BILBERRIES AND BLUEBERRIES Packed with antioxidants such as anthocyanidins that have protective effects on the eyes and the arteries.

GINGER This has warming properties that are beneficial to the circulation.

OLIVE OIL Rich in monounsaturated fats, making it a healthy alternative to other fats and oils. There is also evidence that it may have a beneficial effect on the cardiovascular system.

WATER Perhaps the most important nutrient of all! Hydration is essential for all aspects of health, from digestion to brain function and energy. Many people lose touch with their thirst sensors as they get older, so you need to make it a habit. Start the day with warm water or a herbal tea. Aim to drink seven to eight glasses or mugs of water or herbal tea a day. Avoid drinking too much with meals as this can interfere with proper digestion. Drink before you eat or take little sips during the meal if you need to.

NETTLE TEA Rich in minerals including calcium and iron. It was traditionally used to treat disorders of the muscles, joints and bones, such as arthritis. It is also good for the digestive system. I find it to be a fantastic pick-me-up in the middle of the day. My favourite tea by far.

Foods to avoid

SUGAR Including refined carbohydrates (white bread, white rice, white pasta) and processed foods. These can all upset blood-sugar balance, leading to swings of mood and energy and cravings. They also contribute to tooth decay and are low in nutrients and fibre while being high in calories.

CAFFEINE AND ALCOHOL These affect blood sugar, interfere with sleep, can cause anxiety, raise blood pressure, reduce nutrient status and can be dehydrating, too. Try herbal teas such as rooibos, fennel, peppermint, nettle and chamomile instead.

Top snacks

Smoothies are easy to digest and packed full of nutrients in a form your body can use quickly and easily. Good fruits to put in smoothies include bananas, peaches, pears, apricots, nectarines, berries, avocados and apples.

Rye bread with nut butter – rye bread tends to be easier to digest than wheat bread. Try it lightly toasted with nut or seed butters such as cashew-nut butter or sunflower-seed butter. These provide protein and essential fats.

Avocados are ready to eat when they yield to light pressure. Just cut them in half and eat the flesh with a teaspoon – what a great, tasty source of healthy monounsaturated fats and essential fats!

Bananas are high in potassium needed for a healthy cardiovascular system – plus they're easy to carry with you and eat wherever you are.

Natural soya yoghurt is high in calcium and magnesium as well as phyto-oestrogens. Eat it as it is or stir in some mixed seeds.

Hulled or shelled hemp seeds are soft and easy to chew so can be eaten from the spoon as a healthy pick-me-up – a great source of protein and essential fats.

Olives keep well in the fridge for a few days and provide beneficial fats and the anti-ageing nutrient vitamin E.

- **ADDED SALT** As we age, our sense of taste may decline. This can lead to the temptation to add salt to increase food's flavour. Salt can lead to increased blood pressure and water retention, so use herbs instead. And for those who habitually pour salt onto a meal before they eat it: remember that this meal may have already been laced with salt. The more salt you take in, the more you will need to taste the food. If you feel you must have salt now and again at least use sea salt which is mineralized as opposed to table salt, sodium chloride. But you really don't need to be adding salt at all. You can get fabulous flavour using fresh and dried herbs.

- **CITRUS FRUITS** These can be irritating to the gut for some people, so if you suffer from digestive problems, try replacing them with berries, cherries, apples, pears and apricots instead and see how you feel.

- **WHEAT AND DAIRY PRODUCTS** These can be notoriously hard to digest so avoid challenging the system by using alternative grains such as whole grain, millet, quinoa, amaranth and oat, rice or soya milks.

- **CURED AND PROCESSED MEATS** These are often high in saturated fats (which may be detrimental to cardiovascular health), salt (which can raise blood pressure), and chemical colours, flavourings, preservatives and bulking agents. Avoid bacon, ham, sausages, burgers and the like.

- **TRANS FATS** These are found in some margarines and vegetable fats as well as many processed and fried foods. They are associated with an increased risk of many diseases, including cardiovascular disease. They may appear on food labels as 'hydrogenated' or 'partially hydrogenated' fats or oils.

Recommended supplements

Seek advice from your medical doctor before starting a course of supplements, especially if you are already taking medication.

A good-quality daily multivitamin and mineral complex.

A bone-health formula containing calcium, magnesium, vitamin D, plus other essential bone minerals.

Digestive enzymes with meals.

A daily probiotic for good gut bacteria.

A green superfood to increase your nutrient intake. Easy to digest and packed full of nutrients, examples include blue-green algae, wheat grass, barley grass and spirulina. Chuck them into smoothies or juice; you won't even taste them.

Ginkgo biloba for circulation and brain health.

A fish-oil or flaxseed oil supplement for essential fatty acids, for brain, joint, skin, eye and heart health.

If you're still experiencing hormone-related health issues for the few years post menopause, continue taking whatever supplements or herbs you found helpful to balance them (see previous section on perimenopause, page 225). If you are at all worried about persisting symptoms, do go and see your medical practitioner for further advice.

(For supplements to address specific ailments, see 'Post-menopause and beyond – conditions' section, page 320.)

Daily meal planner

Breakfast: I'm a big fan of oats. They contain soluble fibre that helps to keep cholesterol levels in check and supports healthy digestion, plus they're great for providing sustained energy for several hours. Soak sugar-free and wheat-free muesli overnight in rice or oat milk for a healthy breakfast. Soaking the oats makes them easier to digest. Otherwise, have porridge with a pinch of cinnamon and some vanilla essence. Steel-cut oats are the ones to go for to get that nice long sustained release of energy.

Lunch: It's important not to skip this meal and to get it right in order to avoid energy slumps in the afternoon. Fish, chicken, egg or bean salads, soups, dips and avocados are all good options. Sprinkle nori or kelp flakes onto soups and salads instead of salt for their iodine and mineral content.

Dinner: Eating a big meal late is known to interrupt sleep. You're less active in the evenings so you don't need so much fuel. Soups and salads are light and won't tax your digestion. Otherwise, have baked fish or grilled or poached turkey or chicken, with steamed or roasted vegetables.

Snacks: Good snack foods include fresh or dried fruit, vegetable sticks with dips, avocados, rye bread or oat cakes with nut butter and juices or smoothies. Having a small snack every few hours will keep your blood-sugar levels topped up and your energy and concentration stable.

Food swaps

SWAP: Hot chocolate made with full-fat milk
FOR: Hot 'chocolate' made with rice milk, banana and raw cacao powder

SWAP: White toast with butter and marmalade
FOR: Rye toast with sugar-free jam

SWAP: Three chocolate truffles
FOR: Three soft dried figs

SWAP: Apple pie with custard
FOR: Baked apple with raisins and soya yoghurt

SWAP: Two chocolate biscuits
FOR: Truffles: blend a handful of dates with a few almonds in a food processor. Shape the mixture into balls and roll in raw cacao powder or carob powder.

Some common barriers to good eating

Over the years I've seen enough undernourished clients to build up a good picture of the main reasons why some people don't eat as well as they should. Many of the following won't necessarily apply to you. But they're still well worth reading now, so that you can safeguard against them in the future.

Lack of appetite
It is common for some older people to have a reduced appetite. This may be due to lack of physical activity or poor digestive function. The problem is it can lead to missed meals and poor food choices – you opt for quick, easily digested snacks and convenience foods rather than proper, home-cooked meals.

Lack of daylight
The body manufactures vitamin D through the action of sunlight on the skin. Vitamin D is needed for the utilization of calcium (for strong bones, teeth and nervous function) and is usually low in older people. Yet older women may cover up and stay indoors more than their younger counterparts, especially in winter.

Issues with shopping, preparing food and cooking
Mobility problems in later life can affect what you can buy, how often you go shopping, even what you're able to prepare and cook easily. If you live on your own, you many not feel inclined to cook meals from scratch for yourself. Finances may affect food choices in your retirement years.

Poor chewing and dental problems

If your teeth are starting to deteriorate – you have caps, bridges, false or missing teeth – your ability to chew well may be compromised (a good reason to practise good oral hygiene and see your dentist regularly). Saliva production may also decrease with age. This is significant because optimum digestion starts with the action of chewing and with the enzymes released by saliva in the mouth. Poor digestion can cause discomfort as well as malabsorption of nutrients.

Poor digestive function

Further down the digestive tract, digestion of food depends on the body producing sufficient stomach acid and enzymes. The production of both may decrease with age, so food isn't broken down fully. Side effects include gasiness, bloating, constipation and irregular bowel movements as well as nutrient deficiencies.

Old food habits

There's every chance you have a better diet than people half your age if you were brought up in a time before processed and packaged foods were the norm. But equally this may prevent you taking advantage of the wealth of natural new foods that are now available to us.

As we discussed in the previous chapter on perimenopause, declining oestrogen levels are one of the biggest challenges for women in middle and later life, and can be controlling their waistline. Even if you eat pretty much the same as you always did, the pounds can creep on. As well as the lack of oestrogen, low metabolism can be to blame. The problem is that storing fat around the middle is a risk factor for diabetes and heart disease. It's not good, so you will need to make sure that you eat the right foods to avoid piling on the weight and move that bahookee of yours. Some older women naturally have smaller appetites but it's all about the food choices that you make as to whether or not you will be wearing the effects around your hips and middle. One of the easiest ways to do this? As well as the advice in the previous chapter on avoiding refined carbohydrates and cutting saturated fats and trans fats, simply:

- Always choose lean cuts of meat when you have it and trim off the fat.

- Stick to the simple no-bad-fat cooking methods described above.

- Watch your dairy intake.

- Check the saturated fat and trans hydrogenated fat on all labels.

'For many women the post-menopausal years are wonderful – a time of freedom and joy.'

Feed your brain

One of the biggest worries I hear from women and men alike, from middle age onwards, is that they're losing their marbles. We're hypersensitive about 'senior moments', and panic every time we forget a name, or where we put our mobile, thinking it's a sign of early dementia. Rest assured it's probably not, but you can certainly keep your brain firing by keeping it busy, stimulated and well nourished.

Your brain thrives on plenty of essential fatty acids, antioxidants, zinc, B vitamins and good protein. You also need the steady brain fuel provided by complex carbohydrates and the best nutrient of all, water. (For more on brain health and measures you can take to lessen the risk or slow the progression of Alzheimer's, see page 324).

Some foods for thought

Salmon	Spinach	Amaranth
Tuna	Peas	Millet
Sardines	Pulses	Buckwheat
Chicken	Beans	Oats
Lean white meats	Kelp	Rye
Tempeh	Berries	Barley
Tofu	Brown rice	Nuts and seeds
Eggs	Wheat germ	Curcumin
Avocados	Quinoa	

Supplements for good brain health

Always consult your medical doctor before taking a course
of supplements and, if taking herbs, check with a herbalist
for the correct dosage.

- Liquid algae is rich in protein and amino acids, and may help
  to improve memory, mental clarity and concentration.

- Choline is known as the 'memory vitamin'. Choline enhances
  brain function, mental acuity and neurological systems.

- Lecithin. Two tablespoons of lecithin granules sprinkled
  on your cereal or salad is thought to help restore creativity
  to your thoughts.

- Ginkgo biloba is a herb which may help to improve cognitive
  function.

- Rosemary can help to give that memory a little jog. Spray
  a few drops on a cloth next to your pillow at night.

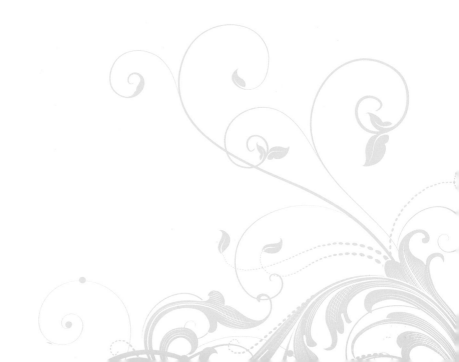

Important lifestyle advice for post-menopause and beyond

Exercising your body – and mind – is vital. It's important for blood-sugar control, normalizing appetite, brain function, mood, energy, joint health, weight and mobility. It can also be a good way to meet other people in your community. Naturally, you need to tailor your exercise to your needs and ability – don't take up a new sport that puts strain on your joints if you have arthritis, for example. Always seek the advice of your doctor. That said I've known people to take up rock climbing in their fifties, jogging in their sixties and salsa in their seventies! Aim for a balance of cardiovascular exercise that gets your heart rate up, and strength-training that works your muscles and joints and protects your bones. Remember, with exercise, it's a case of 'use it or lose it'.

The same goes for your mind – keep those neurons firing. It's never too late to learn a new language, take up another form of study, join a book group. Even doing the daily crossword or Sudoku, or doing mental arithmetic instead of using a calculator will help to keep you mentally sharp.

While teenagers seem to be able to sleep around the clock, later in life quality sleep can be more elusive. In the years around the menopause, hormones and hot flushes can keep us awake at night. Many people also find themselves waking earlier, or not being able to nod off. One explanation may be that you just don't need as much sleep as you used to. If your days are less active, you may need less time to rest and recover. Don't get hung up on numbers – eight hours might be the norm, but if you feel fine after six then don't worry.

Of course, aches and pains, respiratory problems, a weak bladder and other medical conditions can disrupt our slumber. Always have such problems checked out by your

GP if they're interfering with your sleep.

To maximize sleep potential, create the right bedroom environment. Make sure the curtains block out the light properly, and it's not too hot or cold. Wear a night blindfold over your eyes to block out all light. Don't underestimate the value of a decent bed – if yours is over ten years old, it needs replacing. Second, pay attention to what you eat and drink. Avoid caffeine, sugar, rich, salty food, as well as anything more than a tiny tipple of alcohol, late at night. Soporific herbal teas to try instead include chamomile, valerian, lemon balm and hops (but don't drink too much fluid or you'll be waking up to visit the loo!). If you need a pre-bed snack, keep it light – a turkey and lettuce snack would be ideal. Both turkey and lettuce contain natural, sleep-inducing chemicals. You could always opt for my lettuce soup (page 306) earlier in the evening to get you more relaxed.

There's nothing wrong with a mid-afternoon nap if you feel the need and have time. And try to build relaxation into your days so you can switch off better at night. Yoga, meditation, t'ai chi and breathing exercises are all tried and tested ways of managing stress but even listening to some gentle music or going for a walk would be good.

BUT for the best zzzzzzzs . . . GET MOVING. Unless you have a disability or joint issue that prevents you from exercising, do not use advancing years as a reason not to move. You have got to find a way to stay active if you want to nod off at night and sleep deeply. You may no longer be twenty-one but that does not mean that you should stop moving. The more you move that bahookee of yours during the day, the better you will feel and the deeper you will sleep. Make this a mantra of yours: 'I promise to move my bahookee every day as much as I can.' Find a fun exercise and get darn well moving each and every day. That's an order! You'll thank me for it.

Lettuce soup

SERVES 4–6
Suitable for freezing
1 tbsp sunflower or olive oil
1 large onion, peeled and chopped
1 garlic clove, peeled and crushed
450g potatoes, peeled and cut into 2cm pieces
1 litre cold water
2 tbsp wheat-free vegetable stock powder or
   2 vegetable stock cubes
125g millet
1 large romaine lettuce

1 Heat the oil in a large saucepan and fry the onion and garlic over a gentle heat for 5 mins, stirring occasionally. Add the potatoes and cook for 2 mins more.

2 Stir in the water, stock and millet. Bring to the boil and simmer for 15 mins, stirring occasionally. Separate the lettuce into leaves and remove any tough stalks. Roughly shred the remaining leaves and wash in a colander under cold running water.

3 Stir the lettuce into the pan and cover with a lid. Simmer for 3 mins until well wilted, stirring once or twice. Cool in the pan for 5 mins then blend using a hand blender or whiz in a liquidizer until smooth.

4 Return to the pan if necessary and stir in enough cold water to reach a creamy soup consistency – about 300ml/ 1/2 pt. Heat through gently and serve in bowls or mugs.

Lettuce wraps with cashew dressing

SERVES 2

1 medium carrot, peeled and coarsely grated or shredded
1 red pepper, deseeded and finely sliced
2 spring onions, trimmed, halved and finely sliced
75g plain cashew nuts, roughly chopped
75g beansprouts, rinsed
2 romaine lettuces or 1 iceberg lettuce
2–3 tbsp wheat-free tamari soy sauce
For the dressing
3 tbsp tahini (sesame seed paste)
1½ tbsp cider vinegar
3 tbsp cold water

1 To make the dressing, mix all the ingredients in a small bowl with a teaspoon until smooth and creamy-looking.

2 To make the wraps, put all the ingredients, except the lettuce, in small bowls or arrange on a large platter. Remove the six largest leaves from the lettuce and wash. Pat dry with kitchen paper. (Return remaining lettuce to the fridge and use for salads or soup.)

3 Tear one of the leaves in half along the central vein and place one half on top of the other in the palm of your hand. Carefully fill with some of the carrots, pepper, spring onions, nuts and beansprouts. Spoon over a little of the dressing and roll the lettuce firmly around the filling.

4 Cut in half and secure each piece with a cocktail stick if not eating immediately. Put on a large serving plate. Repeat with remaining leaves and fillings. Serve with a small dish of soy sauce for dipping. Remove cocktail sticks before eating.

Gillian's tip: Prepare ahead and serve as a starter or light lunch. These wraps are also great for packed lunches. Try some of your own fillings, too – chopped cooked chicken or flaked tuna make good alternatives to the cashew nuts.

A word (or two) about sex . . .

Let me share a secret about my in-laws. They were so colourful and this is a perfect place to tell you a wee bit about them!

When my mother-in-law was seventy-three and my father-in-law seventy-six, he had congestive heart failure. He lived to tell the tale though. Several years later, I learned that his cardiac arrest actually occurred during sexual relations.

My point is that they were living, loving proof that desires and needs don't need to stop just because you're no longer fertile. The media may not often portray it, but here's the truth: women in their fifties, sixties, seventies and eighties can be highly sexual beings. They're as capable of having orgasms as women in their twenties, years of experience have taught them what they like and how to get it.

Now you may be reading this and nodding furiously, thinking, That's me, that's me! Or perhaps you're thinking, That should be me, but my body won't co-operate. Or maybe you're more of a 'thanks, but no thanks' woman. Well, all of the above are normal. It's your body and your sex life and you can have as much or as little as you like.

Your post-menopausal years can be a fantastic time to have sex. You don't have to worry about getting pregnant (although it's a good idea to carry on using contraception for a year after you think you've gone through the menopause. And if you have a new partner, you still need to use condoms to protect against STIs), periods and in some cases the kids walking in; some of you may still worry about that.

You may, however, need to make some modifications. Natural lubrication may be in short supply, or your libido may fluctuate – there are plenty of remedies for such issues (see 'Low libido', page 377). Many women report orgasms post-menopause being more of a full-body experience. But if you and your partner are happy not having sex very often, or at all, that's absolutely fine, too. Intimacy and love can be shown in many ways, so take time each day to show affection, hold hands and hug.

Health checks, screening and diagnostic tests

Your risk of illness increases in later life, so it's important to keep a close check on yourself. This means a combination of self-awareness and being proactive about visiting your GP, attending the regular screenings you're invited for on the NHS and perhaps organizing additional diagnostic tests. Please don't be dismayed by the list that follows – they're simply precautions. We're lucky that so many conditions are detectable at such an early stage when they can often be prevented, reversed or treated more successfully.

Self-checks

You know yourself and your body better than anyone else, and now more than ever you need to be aware of any changes that don't seem normal for you. That could be significant changes in your mood, your energy levels, your appetite, your weight. It could be any unusual lumps, pains, skin changes, a persistent cough, visual disturbances, unusual vaginal or rectal bleeding or changes to your normal bowel habits. Rest assured they are probably nothing serious. Nonetheless make a note and report them to your GP.

Breast awareness

Your home health MOT should include regular breast checks. These days, cancer experts don't advise a set routine or frequency for doing this, they just suggest you become familiar with how your breasts normally look and feel (and how this might change over the course of a month, if you're still having periods or recently post-menopausal). Fix a regular time to do this, such as the start of each month.

Look at your breasts in a mirror; see how they feel when you're lying down, and standing, and when your arms are raised over your head. Note their size, shape, colour, what your nipples look like. Touch your breasts and all around them, from your armpits to your collarbone and get used to how they normally feel – breasts can be dense and lumpy at the best of times.

What you're checking for are any changes such as lumps, swellings, or bulging of breast tissue; any dimples or puckering of the skin, redness, pain or inflammation, changes to the shape or position of your nipples or discharge from them.

Remember that the vast majority of lumps reported turn out to be benign – but also that the majority of cancers are first detected by the woman herself or her partner.

NHS screening

When you are over the age of forty, your GP should perform regular cardiovascular risk checks, in which they look at your weight, age, family and smoking history, blood sugars, blood cholesterol levels and blood pressure to build an overall picture of your heart health and to see if you need more frequent monitoring. If you're not invited for this roughly every two years, make an appointment and ask.

Every five years you'll be asked to attend your cervical smear test, until the age of sixty-four. After this age you can request them. You can also have a pelvic examination at the same time if this is something that you feel you need.

Between the ages of fifty and seventy, you'll be invited for a mammogram – an X-ray of the breasts – to screen for breast cancer every three years (again, you can request them after this age if you're worried). In recent years, this type of screening has attracted some controversy. Some people believe the radiation and compression involved may actually increase risk or exacerbate an existing cancer. Ultimately, the choice is yours but it's clear the NHS still believes they're a valid and important screening tool.

When you're over the age of sixty (fifty in Scotland and Wales), you'll be sent a stool test (called a faecal occult blood test) by post every two years to check for early signs of bowel cancer by looking for blood in your stool sample. You can request this earlier (or have it privately) if you're worried about symptoms or a family history of bowel disorders. Screening continues until you're sixty-nine, but you can request a test after this age.

Although it's entirely up to you whether you take part in any of these screening programmes, I think it's important to realize that they're offered to us because GPs know they work. Think how drastically underfunded we're always hearing the NHS is – a national screening programme would not be in place if it hadn't been proved that a particular form of screening enables early detection, and that early detection saves lives. Bowel cancer (screening through stool tests) is a perfect example of a cancer that, if detected early enough, is a life saver in more than 90 per cent of cases.

Other tests

It's up to you to make sure you visit your dentist and optometrist at least every two years – more, of course, if you experience problems with your teeth or eyes.

Bone density

There are various tests available for measuring bone density and bone turnover, designed to measure your risk of osteoporosis, fracture and, sometimes, other bone disorders. The risk of osteoporosis fractures increases every seven years after the age of fifty. So you must do everything possible to protect and nourish your skeletal structure (see page 227). Your GP may recommend you have them if you are at risk of osteoporosis or have a family history of the disease, have fractured a bone after a modest trauma, use steroid medications or are pre-menopausal but very thin and have not had a period for a number of years. It's worth asking if you're concerned, or you can also pay to have the tests privately at many health clinics. Home-testing kits you can buy from chemists, health-food shops and online tend to be urine tests that measure the rate at which bone is being broken down. This will tell you the rate of bone loss but does not give an indication of new bone formation or current density. To find out the current status of your bone density a DEXA scan is generally recommended. This stands for Dual Energy X-ray Absorptiometry and can detect more information about the health of the bones than normal X-rays. Large, free-standing DEXA machines are used to measure the density of the hip or lower spine, while small, portable devices are used to measure the density of the wrist, finger or heel. It takes about twenty minutes and is entirely painless. The scan creates a picture of your bones, showing the bone density. A computer then compares your bone density against the norm for your age and size. This gives an indication of your risk of fracture. Other tests to measure bone density include dual photon absorptiometry and computed tomography scans.

Homocysteine test

For many years, the measurement of cholesterol levels in the blood has been seen as the clearest indicator of heart and cardiovascular problems. More recently it has been discovered that raised levels of 'homocysteine' may also be indicative of potential problems. Research shows that a three-point decrease in homocysteine levels reduces the risk of heart attacks by up to 16 per cent, strokes by 24 per cent and deep vein thrombosis by 25 per cent.

Excess homocysteine becomes toxic and begins to damage and thicken artery walls, as well as causing blood to clot more readily. Levels above normal have been found in 30–40 per cent of patients with early cardiovascular disease. Elevated levels can also interfere with the synthesis of other vital substances, such as hormones and antioxidants. This then creates other problems throughout the body. Your homocysteine level may predict your susceptibility to risk for more than 100 medical conditions including cardiovascular disease, diabetes, arthritis and Alzheimer's disease among others.

You may be at risk of high homocysteine if you:
- Eat an unhealthy diet
- Do not take regular exercise
- Are overweight
- Smoke
- Drink excessive amounts of coffee or alcohol

- Have been diagnosed with cardiovascular problems such as high cholesterol or high blood pressure.

If your GP does not offer you a homocysteine test it is possible to have a test done privately (see www.gillianmckeith.info).

The stool test

As well as the faecal occult stool test offered on the NHS (which simply checks for blood in stools), it is possible to have a more thorough test done privately, for a better picture of your overall bowel health. If you have any of the following classic signs of an unhealthy gut and ineffective digestion, you'd benefit from a test:

- A full or bloated feeling in your stomach, especially after eating
- Regular occurrences of wind/flatulence
- Loose stools (diarrhoea) or constipation
- A reluctance to eat certain foods because they make you feel uncomfortable
- Abdominal cramps or pains
- Ongoing chronic infections or chronic fatigue
- A feeling that your bowels have not been 'right' since suffering a bout of food poisoning
- Taken antibiotics for more than one month at a time, or taken oral contraceptives, HRT or steroids for extended periods

Stool tests are generally used to detect pathogenic bacteria, yeasts, parasites, worms or the presence of undigested foods. Tests can be carried out in the comfort of your own home, without the need to go to a clinic or visit a specialist. Everything you need to carry out the test is sent to you with full instructions detailing how to carry out the test (see www.gillianmckeith.info).

The pelvic examination

Pelvic examinations are available for women of menopausal age and beyond. It is something that could be done every one to three years if you want, depending on your personal health history and family history. You can ask if your GP (or a Well Woman Clinic) will do this for you when you book to attend your cervical smear test. Or you could see a private medical doctor. During the examination the medical doctor will gently evaluate the size and position of your vagina, cervix, uterus, ovaries, Fallopian tubes, bladder and rectum. They will use lubrication and gloves and try to make you as comfortable as possible. The main aim is to detect possible cancers, infections, sexually transmitted infections, fibroids, cysts, prolapses and other gynaecological problems. The earlier these conditions are detected, the easier they are to treat.

Post-menopause energy synchronization

Menopausal symptoms are simply an indication of energy change, a rebalancing in your body. This is not necessarily a time of energy loss, but rather energy transformation. It is the phase of your life that can potentially open the body, mind and spirit to a new vibrational flow with wondrous possibilities to explore and to fully discover the self. This is a most exciting time to create your own reality for your life.

In private practice, I have consulted with many female clients who were going through post-menopause and reported experiencing feelings of depression, the blues or just the 'blahs'. They told me that they did not feel attractive, that they were 'invisible' and felt irrelevant. I am here to tell you that these feelings are incorrect, made up and nothing more than a 'head game' that you don't need. Instead, calm your mind, go into the body; feel who you really are. You are not a compilation of superfluous wants: wanting jewellery, wanting money, wanting approval, wanting men to desire you, wanting a large house, wanting sex appeal, wanting material things. There is nothing inherently wrong with wanting things, but it doesn't define the foundation of anyone. In a sense it's a mind game played with yourself. At your core, you are none of this.

As a result of your life experience, you now are in a powerful position to explore your own truth, peace and purpose. You can decide that this is the prime of your life as you are at the height of your wisdom, self-discovery and self-awareness. It is about shifting from negative to positive. When you clear your mind of all the chatter, you can hear and feel the real you – what you really feel in your heart, not what someone else tells you to think.

This is your chance to take responsibility for creating your own harmonized reality. We can decide to listen to the thoughts and directives of others, whether teachers, spouses, clergymen, parents, friends, journalists, politicians, corporates or whoever, and decide that their values, beliefs and thoughts are the culmination of who we are; or we can simply feel our own selves and our own sensations, our own feelings, and our own true wants. Once you delve and discover the real you rather than the society-created version of your self, then you will find and note the difference.

In effect, this is the time to find your real self. I view post-menopause as the culmination of a woman's discovery of life: the pinnacle of wisdom, inner exploration, spiritual awareness and focus of the self; not for selfish reasons, but for selfless reasons. When you find your inner peace, you then bring harmony to those around you and ultimately you contribute to the balance of the whole world. Take the reins and then this period of life promises to be the culmination of who you really are. You can finally discover, express and manifest the full you. This is the purpose of your life.

To help you to focus and manifest your highest self at this period of your life, I would like you to play with a few key energy regions, especially an area sometimes referred to as the sixth chakra or 'the third eye', located just above the nose between the eyebrows, though ever so slightly above. This is a vibrational region of your body for developing your creativity, meditation, intuition and your connection with yourself as well as your connection with all energies within and outside yourself and beyond. In other words, by strengthening this specific energy centre, you can better find your true self. Other key energy regions are the solar plexus and the heart. So here we go:

Five-step energy balancing

1   Lie down in a comfortable position (on a mat or bed) in a quiet room and close your eyes.

2   Listen to your breath. Let your body do the breathing; you don't need to force the breath. Instead, imagine you can see your breath coming into your whole body, filling your feet and legs, tummy, chest, back, arms, neck, head; and then imagine you see the breath going out of your body. Watch the inhalations and exhalations for about a minute.

3   Once relaxed, imagine a ball of white (or yellow) light swirling around your solar plexus or tummy region; and a ball of white (or green) light swirling around your chest or heart region. Visualize it for about one minute.

4   Now go to the region just above your nose between your eyebrows. Imagine a swirling ball of white light (or pastel purple or pale indigo) in this energy region. The visualized light illuminates as you imagine this light growing, getting bigger in your head, and eventually taking over your whole body and even the room. Just bathe yourself in this light.

5   Now lie there and continue to listen to the breath and feel or visualize the light throughout every part of your body and soul. Just be with it.

This five-step process for energy balancing need not take you more than about five minutes to do.

A few other tips to balance post-menopausal energy:

> **FOODS** Supportive foods include sweet vegetables such as roasted squash, pumpkin, sweet potatoes, carrots, oats, sea vegetables, yoghurt, miso, vanilla seeds and pods, cinnamon and sweet cicely, aubergine, purple cabbage, blackberries and all green vegetables. Use vanilla seeds and pods, cinnamon and sweet cicely instead of sugar.

> **TEAS** Drink nettle, sage and oat-straw teas for their specific nourishing properties.

> **CREATE** Sing, dance, write, paint, sketch, draw, get involved in community charity, start a new business or project, enrol on a course, take up a musical instrument, knit. (Note: There is nothing 'old-fogey' about knitting or sewing. My ten-year-old daughter loves it and seems to get all meditative when she's doing it! She asked me the other day to teach her how to crochet.)

> **BOOGIE** Physically freeing the body is so very important; dancing and other moderate but regular fitness exercises are ideal. Let go and boogie at every opportunity, every day. Belly-dancing is fantastic – find a class and wiggle that sacral centre! But if group gyrating isn't your cup of tea (although you should give it a go . . . it's great fun), just stand with your feet hip-width apart and circle your hips in each direction, then make a figure of eight in each direction. But any form of dance is great: hip-hop, street dance, flamenco, jazz, ballroom, ballet – take your pick. Also check out t'ai chi and yoga; they are both good exercises for improving energy flow throughout the body. They also build strength, balance and flexibility which are important aspects of staying healthy. Try swimming, Pilates (my favourite), chi gung, walking, stretching and anything else that gets you moving.

Post-menopause and beyond – conditions

Age-related macular degeneration

Age-related macular degeneration (AMD) is so called because it's most common in people over sixty. In fact it's the leading cause of blindness in people over fifty-five in the West and women are more prone to it than men. It's characterized by a gradual or sudden loss of central and detailed vision. There are two types, wet and dry.

In wet AMD, the small blood vessels that supply the back of the eye (the macula) start to swell and leak. This causes scarring that leads to blurring and eventually a blind spot, right in the centre of your vision. Wet macular degeneration is much less common than dry and is characterized by new blood vessels developing under the retina causing haemorrhaging and swelling with the development of scar tissue. Wet macular degeneration tends to develop quickly and has a more severe effect on the central vision.

The most common type of AMD is dry macular degeneration. This is caused by a build-up of waste products, called drusen, beneath the retina and is characterized by loss of pigment in the retina. Dry macular degeneration usually progresses slowly over years. At the moment there is no known treatment to cure the disease.

AMD sometimes only causes a slight distortion of vision. However, for some people, it ends up with a total loss of central vision where even reading and driving become impossible. It does not affect the peripheral vision so does not cause total blindness.

Symptoms
- Blurring in the centre of your vision
- Reduced visual acuity e.g. difficulty distinguishing faces
- Distortion of straight lines – they may appear wavy or bent
- Poor colour vision
- Need for better lighting
- Reduced night vision
- Blind spots in your central vision – these appear as dark patches or empty spaces

What you can do

Unfortunately, there is currently no treatment for dry AMD. Treatment for wet AMD is usually with lasers or injections to seal off the leaking blood vessels and slow the progression of the disease. It's far from satisfactory, as it can't actually cure AMD and some of the healthy cells may be destroyed in the process. The plus side, however, is that there's plenty you can do to prevent the condition from developing – or slow its progression if you've already been diagnosed.

AMD is strongly linked to free-radical damage caused by smoking, exposure to UV light and a diet lacking in antioxidants. Make sure you always wear good-quality sunglasses in bright light. Look for the CE or UV400 marks as a guarantee of quality, and choose larger styles for proper coverage (think Jackie O, not John Lennon!).

Not smoking and avoiding exposure to second-hand smoke are obviously key. But perhaps most important is to really fill up on brightly coloured, antioxidant-rich fruit and veggies. Carotenoids called lutein and xeazanthin are the key antioxidants for eye health. You'll find them in yellow and green veg.

It goes without saying that you should always attend

check-ups with your optometrist – at least every two years. It doesn't matter if you don't wear spectacles or lenses, or have symptoms – optometrists have the training and equipment needed to spot eye conditions at a very early stage.

If you start to experience any of the above symptoms, it's important to get them checked out by an optometrist straight away as the earlier AMD is diagnosed the better the outcome in the future. If you notice any of your friends or relatives having vision problems, suggest they go for a check-up. You may notice they are having trouble seeing in dim light or they might shut one eye to focus more clearly.

A quick test
Cover one eye and focus on a door frame or other straight line. If it appears wavy, then get yourself to the optometrist as you may have the early stages of macular degeneration.

Gillian's diet and supplement tips
Always consult a medical doctor before taking a course of supplements.

> Lutein and zeaxanthin are part of the pigment of the macular. Evidence suggests that they help to slow the development and progression of the disease. Some of the best sources of these antioxidants are kale, turnip greens, spinach and broccoli.

> Eat plenty of carotenoid-rich green leafy and yellow fruit and veg. Think spinach, kale, apricots, nectarines.

> Berries are also high in eye-protective flavonoids – bilberries and blueberries contain anthocyanins that have antioxidant effects as well as the ability to strengthen capillaries and peripheral circulation.

- Eat oily fish, for their protective omega-3 fats, good for general eye health.

- Zinc is another eye-friendly nutrient. Find it in abundance in pumpkin seeds and raw shelled hemp seeds, too.

- Vitamin E has antioxidant properties that may help to protect the eye from damage. Good sources include almonds, seeds, olives, avocados, wheatgerm and cold-pressed sesame oil and olive oil.

- High blood pressure increases AMD risk, so avoid sugar, refined foods, alcohol, caffeine, burnt or fried foods, heated fats.

- People who are overweight are more likely to develop AMD so if you are overweight, take steps to lose the excess flab now.

- Move that body of yours with regular exercise – this improves your circulation which has a protective effect on the eyes.

- Make sure you always wear good-quality sunglasses in bright light. Look for the CE or UV400 marks as a guarantee of quality, and choose larger styles for proper coverage.

- If you smoke, give up as soon as possible and avoid exposure to second-hand smoke.

- My top supplements for good eye health are: taurine, lutein, lycopene, zeaxanthin, ginkgo and bilberry.

Coping with the symptoms

- Buy big – large-print books, large-number telephones, watches with large numbers – all these are available.

- Use contrasting colours – a dark-coloured cup on a white tablecloth stands out.

- Use a magnifying glass.

- Work or read near the window during daylight hours or in well-lit rooms.

- Shine the light directly onto what you are reading.

- Consult a low-vision specialist – these professionals can recommend equipment and techniques that can help to improve your quality of life.

Alzheimer's disease

Alzheimer's is a degenerative brain disease that affects women more than men. It's the most common type of dementia in the UK – and one that many folks express fear of developing. It's important to emphasize here that Alzheimer's is *not* an inevitable consequence of ageing. The vast majority (about 90 per cent) of those over eighty have no symptoms of the disease at all.

It is often difficult to diagnose Alzheimer's in the early stages. The distressing symptoms include memory (particularly short-term memory) loss and confusion. As time goes on there may be problems finding the right words for objects, names and places. Speech and understanding can be compromised. Those with Alzheimer's may understandably experience mood swings and feel angry, irritable, apathetic, frustrated, scared and sad. They often increasingly withdraw from social events, probably due to failure to recognize people or finding communication difficult. As the disease progresses, they may be unable to carry out simple tasks unaided, such as making a cup of tea or warming up a can of soup – they may forget the stages involved or forget they have put the pan on the cooker. Judgement may become compromised, affecting awareness of danger. Alzheimer's can alter a person's intellectual capacity to the point where simple daily tasks become impossible.

So what causes Alzheimer's? The symptoms are caused by the death of nerve cells in the brain and a shortage of neurotransmitters which are responsible for sending messages around the brain and nervous system. Those with Alzheimer's have an accumulation of plaques and tangles, known as amyloid plaques and tau tangles, in the brain. It is not known whether these cause the disease or are a symptom of it. The loss of connections in the parts of the brain dealing with short-term memory often causes the initial symptoms. The disease progresses and spreads, gradually affecting cells in other parts of the brain.

Alzheimer's is a complex disease and no single factor has yet been proven as the single cause of the disease. It is likely that in each case many factors play a part in the onset and speed of progression. Some of these factors are out of our control but others may be mitigated by our diet or lifestyle.

Risk factors
Being over sixty-five, female and having a genetic predisposition to the disease are known to increase risk. Other factors that may contribute include smoking, a previous severe head injury and having high blood pressure. Although not proven, there are some suggestions that your environment and general health can be contributory factors. There is also debate over a potential link between heavy metal poisoning (exposure to cadmium, aluminium, mercury) and Alzheimer's.

Feed your brain and memory

Mackerel with pine nuts and parsley

SERVES 2
2 mackerel, cleaned and filleted
For the filling
2 spring onions, trimmed and finely sliced
3 tbsp pine nuts, roughly chopped
3 tbsp fresh chopped parsley
Finely grated rind of 1 lemon
1 garlic clove, peeled and finely chopped
Mixed salad leaves, tomatoes, cucumber,
  sliced peppers, to serve
Lemon wedges, for squeezing

1 Preheat the grill to medium-hot. Line a grill pan with foil. Mix the spring onions, pine nuts, parsley, lemon rind and garlic together in a small bowl.

2 Slash the mackerel twice on each side then open out, skin side down. Spoon the filling down the middle of each mackerel. Bring the sides up to enclose the filling and place the fish on the grill pan.

3 Grill for 5 minutes on each side until cooked through and lightly browned. Serve on a large bed of mixed salad with fresh lemon wedges for squeezing.

4 Serve with purple sprouting broccoli and baked squash. The mackerel provides the essential fats needed for brain function. The vegetables supply antioxidants needed to protect the brain from damage.

General lifestyle tips

- It's vital to keep your brain active throughout life – learn a new language, do crossword puzzles or Sudoku, take up tango lessons . . . Stay mentally and socially active.

- Keep stress at bay. The stress hormone cortisol has a negative effect on brain function so don't give your brain an acid bath by flooding it with stress hormones.

- Take regular exercise – physical activity is also known to reduce dementia risk (as well as reducing stress levels and boosting mood).

- Ask a holistic dentist to check your mercury fillings for leakage and possible replacement.

- When cooking, I would prefer you to use stainless steel, ceramic and glass cookware.

- Traces of aluminium may be found in processed cheeses, pickles, cake mixes, baking soda and some processed foods, so read the labels.

- Avoid deodorants, douches, shampoos and medicines such as antacids that contain aluminium.

- Investigate chelation therapy. This is a procedure that involves intravenous infusions of a substance called EDTA as well as minerals. It can help to remove heavy metals from the system. Well worth it. To find out more, contact the Arterial Disease Clinic.

Bowel cancer

Bowel cancer is the second most common cancer in women (after breast cancer) so it's something that should definitely be on your radar. One in twenty people are diagnosed at some stage in their lives, and each year there are over 36,000 new cases in the UK.

Also known as colon or colorectal cancer, it's a malignant disease of the large bowel (colon) or rectum. The good news is survival rates are improving, and if caught early enough the disease is highly treatable.

Causes and risk factors

- It's thought about two-thirds of cases of bowel cancer could have been prevented by dietary changes. Of particular risk is a diet low in fibre, fruit and veg and high in meat and saturated fat.

- Your risk increases the older you are. About 85 per cent of cases are in people over sixty. But it's on the increase in younger people and, for prevention and early detection reasons, you must be aware now.

- If you have a strong family history of bowel cancer (that's a first-degree relative affected before the age of forty-five, or two at any age), breast or ovarian cancer, or bowel polyps, your risk is increased.

- A history of inflammatory bowel disorders such as Crohn's disease or ulcerative colitis, or polyps also increases risk.

- If you regularly consume alcohol, especially beer; smoke; are inactive or overweight or obese, you're putting yourself at risk.

Warning signs to look out for

- Persistent changes in bowel habits that aren't normal for you, such as loose stools for several weeks
- Bleeding from the bottom
- Blood in the stools
- Abdominal discomfort or pain
- A lump in the abdomen
- Extreme tiredness with no known cause
- Unexplained weight loss

Don't be too embarrassed to speak up. These symptoms may not indicate that you have bowel cancer but it is best to get checked. The problem is that many of these symptoms can indicate other less serious digestive problems so they often go unreported. Some people don't see their GP until they experience one of the final three symptoms on the list – by which time if it's cancer, it may be more advanced.

So always report any changes in your bowel habit to your GP. Look behind you when you go to the loo – check what comes out and look at the paper after you've wiped. Don't be squeamish, this is your health and life we're talking about!

After sixty, you'll routinely be invited to give stool samples for a faecal occult blood test on the NHS which screens for signs of bowel cancer (see page 314). But if you have any of the risk factors mentioned above, ask your GP about early screening. Check out: beatingbowelcancer.org.

What you can do

Diet and lifestyle changes can have a massive impact on your chances of preventing the disease – and, indeed, recovering well if you've been diagnosed. Stress relief is important so you will need to take time out for you. It's absolutely essential that you stop smoking, lose weight if you need to and take regular exercise. If you are being treated for bowel cancer, make sure you check with your GP before taking any of my suggested supplements or starting up exercise.

Gillian's diet tips

› A high-fibre diet aids regular bowel movements and provides protection against bowel cancer. Opt for whole grain cereals such as brown rice, millet, quinoa and amaranth. Avoid refined (white) grains as they've had their fibre removed. Other excellent sources include beans and pulses, vegetables, fruit and sprouted beans and seeds.

› When it comes to fresh fruit and vegetables, make five-a-day your absolute minimum. If possible, I want you to aim for seven to nine portions a day. Besides being a good source of fibre, these food groups are abundant in phytonutrients – powerful plant antioxidants that have anti-cancer activity.

› Freshly pressed fruit and vegetable juices are a fantastic way to up your antioxidant intake, detoxify and supercharge the body.

› Cruciferous veggies – like broccoli, cauliflower, Brussels sprouts, cabbage and kale – contain several cancer-protective substances including indole-3-carbinol, glucaric acid and sulforaphane. Research suggests people who eat them regularly have a reduced risk of bowel cancer.

› Tomatoes contain a phytonutrient called lycopene, consumption of which has been associated with a reduced risk of bowel cancer. It's better absorbed from cooked tomatoes rather than raw, so grilled or baked tomatoes with a little extra virgin olive oil would be ideal. Even tomato sauces or tinned tomatoes count as a source of lycopene, but do beware the sugar content as it can be deceptively high.

> Include garlic, preferably raw, in your diet often. It's been found to lower the risk of bowel cancer, which may be due to its ability to reduce the development of cancer-forming compounds in the body.

> To fight constipation, drink plenty of water. It'll help keep the motions soft and moving through the colon. Drink at least eight glasses of bottled or filtered water daily. Herbal teas are good, too – I like nettle and dandelion teas for their detoxifying, bowel-moving and fortifying abilities.

> You're going to have to cut right back on – ideally eliminate – meat, especially red. Processed meat products in particular are most definitely linked with bowel cancer – so please, no sausages, hams, pies, and the like. Well-done or charred meat (typical BBQ fare) contains more cancer-forming compounds than lightly cooked meat. People with bowel cancer should avoid meat altogether and eat other sources of protein instead, such as tofu, beans, whole grains, quinoa, nuts, seeds, eggs (no more than five a week), fish and natural live yoghurt.

> Avoid foods high in saturated fat such as full-fat dairy products (butter, cream and cheese), as well as foods that contain toxic trans fats such as hard margarine, biscuits and anything that has been deep-fried.

> Cut out alcohol and caffeinated drinks including coffee and black tea. Instead, drink grain coffee substitutes, green tea which contains an antioxidant compound called epigallocatechin gallate (EGCG), and herbal teas such as fennel, chamomile, peppermint, ginger and rooibos.

Supplement and herb tips

Always consult your medical doctor before taking a course of supplements and a herbalist for the correct dosage of herbs.

- Vitamin C has been demonstrated to reduce the risk of bowel cancer in women.

- Some studies have shown that people who take vitamin E supplements may have a decreased risk of pre-cancerous colon polyps and bowel cancer, probably due to the vitamin's antioxidant effect.

- Blood levels of the antioxidant mineral selenium have been found to be low in people with bowel cancer and other cancers, so I'd advise a supplement. It also appears to boost immune function in bowel cancer patients.

- Studies have found that people who eat more garlic have a lower incidence of bowel cancer, so taking it in supplement form as well as eating more may be worthwhile.

- Reishi mushroom can be taken in capsule form for its anti-cancer and immune-boosting effects.

- Salvestrols are natural plant compounds that researchers believe may trigger a protein in our cells that could halt the progression of cancer. They're found in fruit and vegetables but as modern farming methods have depleted their levels, you may like to take a salvestrol supplement.

- IP-6 is a compound present in oat and wheat bran that you can also take in supplement form. Studies show it has anti-cancer properties, especially in relation to bowel cancer.

Cardiovascular disease

Heart disease is often thought of as a man's disease, yet it's the number one cause of death in women – killing more of us than breast cancer. After the age of fifty, the risk of heart disease in women increases dramatically, because the protective effect of oestrogen is lost. Women who have an early menopause, either naturally or surgically induced, are also at greater risk.

Cardiovascular disease (CVD) is an umbrella term for heart problems which may include conditions such as coronary heart disease (CHD), congestive heart failure, cardiomyopathy, cerebral vascular disease, stroke, carotid artery disease, atherosclerosis, arteriosclerosis and peripheral vascular disease.

The cardiovascular system comprises the heart and the veins, arteries and capillaries. The heart is a muscle that is responsible for pumping the blood around the body. The blood is carried to and from the heart by the arteries, arterioles, capillaries and veins. The cardiovascular system also carries water, nutrients, salts and waste products to and from the cells.

CVD is generally caused by a lack of blood flow to the arteries supplying the heart, carotid arteries, brain or legs. This can result from atherosclerosis, a build-up of plaque which leads to a lack of oxygen supplying the organs of the body. Common symptoms can include chest pain, skipped or irregular heartbeats, shortness of breath, high blood pressure, dizzy spells and pain in the jaw or legs.

Risk factors for developing CVD

- Genetic predisposition
- High blood pressure
- High cholesterol – specifically high LDL cholesterol and/or low HDL cholesterol
- High homocysteine levels (an amino acid, high blood levels of which are a strong marker for CVD and CHD – see page 313)
- Smoking
- Diabetes
- Being overweight/obese – especially carrying extra weight around the middle
- A sedentary lifestyle
- A poor diet, high in trans fats and saturated fats
- Hormonal imbalances
- Gum disease
- High levels of the inflammatory marker CRP (ask your GP about this)
- Bacterial imbalances
- Exposure to lead and heavy metals
- Inflammatory conditions such as rheumatoid arthritis
- Hormone-replacement therapy.

In the past, HRT was thought to reduce the risk of heart disease. However, some trials have reported that there may in fact be an increase in the risk of cardiovascular heart disease, especially in the first year after starting HRT. In 2002 the Women's Health Initiative trial looked at the effect of HRT on thousands of healthy post-menopausal women. They found an increased risk of heart disease, stroke and thrombosis in women using HRT, compared with those who were not.

For many women, having a heart attack is their first indication of a problem with the cardiovascular system. Although, on investigation, most sufferers had previous symptoms without realizing what they might mean. If you experience any of the following, see your GP:

- Unexplained fatigue or sleep problems
- Mood changes – irritability, depression, insomnia and anxiety
- Indigestion or nausea
- Pressure or pain in the chest, stomach, back or neck
- Headaches
- Shortness of breath
- Rapid heartbeat, palpitations or an irregular heartbeat
- Visual disturbances or light-headedness
- Cold sweats

What you can do

Everyone over forty should see their GP regularly for a cardiovascular check, which will assess their risk based on weight, age, family history, cholesterol, blood pressure and blood sugars. It's also a good idea to ask for your homocysteine levels to be checked.

Because there's a huge lifestyle component to CVD, there's a great deal you can do to both prevent it and to improve your recovery rate if you already have symptoms. Smoking, for a start, doubles your risk of developing heart disease. Second-hand smoke also increases your risk. Being overweight is a major risk factor, but the following dietary and exercise advice will help with that.

It's vital to avoid excess alcohol consumption, and you must limit or eliminate saturated and trans fats, as found in fatty meats, fried foods, high-fat dairy products and any products which contain hydrogenated fats and heated or processed vegetable oils. Become a label reader!

Gillian's diet tips

> Omega-3 fatty acids have been linked to good heart health so up your intake of oily cold-water fish such as salmon, haddock and sardines.

> Diets high in soluble fibre have been shown in some studies to lower total cholesterol and LDL cholesterol. Include in your diet oat bran, beans, raspberries, mustard greens, cauliflower, collard greens, broccoli, chard and turnip greens – all good sources.

> B vitamins are important for normal function of blood vessels and maintaining normal blood pressure. They also help the body to break down homocysteine, a substance which can accumulate and damage blood vessels. Include whole grains, such as quinoa and oats which are a good source of B vitamins, in particular B3, B6 and folic acid.

> Asparagus is rich in vitamin B3 (niacin) which helps to balance the body's production of cholesterol. Other food sources include crimini mushrooms, tuna, chicken, halibut and salmon.

> Cultures in which soy foods constitute a major portion of the diet typically have much lower rates of heart disease than cultures with a low consumption of soy. Soy is a good source of the co-enzyme Q10 which has been shown to lower blood pressure by lowering cholesterol levels and stabilizing the vascular system.

> Numerous studies show regular consumption of garlic may help to lower blood pressure. This is due not only to its sulphur compounds, but its vitamin C, selenium, manganese and also its vitamin B6 content.

Too much sodium can cause the body to retain extra fluid, causing blood pressure to rise. But potassium has a diuretic effect, helping to excrete excess sodium and keep fluid levels and blood pressure in balance. Avoid table salt and up your intake of potassium-rich fruit and veg – bananas are an excellent source.

Drinking cranberry juice may help to increase the 'good' HDL cholesterol levels, probably due to the fruit's high levels of polyphenols – potent antioxidants.

A high intake of magnesium is associated with lower blood pressure and improved cardiovascular health. Get yours from sunflower seeds, pumpkin seeds, brown rice, kale, broccoli, savoy cabbage, rocket, watercress, dulse, kelp, millet, almonds and alfalfa sprouts.

Antioxidants such as flavonoids found in fruit, vegetables and spices such as turmeric have been shown to have a protective effect on the cardiovascular system.

Research has found that eating two kiwi fruits a day can have a protective effect on the cardiovascular system with improved cholesterol ratios. This is likely to be due to the high vitamin C and antioxidant content of kiwi fruits.

Include almonds which, along with sunflower and safflower oils, are a good source of vitamin E. Of all the antioxidants, the fat-soluble antioxidant vitamin E not only reduces LDL (bad) cholesterol but also increases HDL (good) cholesterol levels, and increases the breakdown of fibrin, a clot-forming protein. Other sources of vitamin E include avocados, wheatgerm and cold-pressed sesame oil.

Seek out natto – a fermented soy product similar to miso. It has been found to have heart-protective properties, and is perhaps one of the reasons why Japanese people are less likely to develop heart disease. It's a good way to flavour soups and stews.

- Nettle tea has a slight diuretic effect that may reduce blood pressure and it's also rich in potassium and other heart-helping minerals.

Supplement and herb tips

If you have an existing heart condition or are taking medication (particularly blood-thinning medication), always check with your GP before taking any supplements as there may be a bad reaction. If taking herbs, check with a herbalist for the correct dosage.

- Folic acid is so important for cardiovascular function that one study found 400mcg a day could prevent 28,000 cardiovascular deaths per year.

- Many studies have demonstrated that either fish-oil supplements or flaxseed oil, two great sources of omega-3 essential fats, are effective in lowering blood pressure.

- Red yeast rice extract can lower total cholesterol, LDL and triglycerides (blood lipids or fats) as well as reducing inflammation in the blood vessels. Ask your local health-food store to order it for you if they don't stock it.

- Hawthorn leaf extracts may help to strengthen the heart muscle.

- Ginkgo biloba tea is another powerful cardiovascular helper as it can improve blood circulation.

- Motherwort herbal extract – an excellent all-round heart tonic, especially for women. It is useful for calming palpitations and irregular heartbeats and is useful if stress or anxiety are present. A specialist herbal shop will stock this or ask your local health-food store to order it.

Co-enzyme Q10 is beneficial for various aspects of cardiovascular function. Its levels in the body decline with age. Statins, often given for high cholesterol, lower levels further.

General lifestyle tips

Learn to manage stress – stress can increase blood pressure and the chance of developing cardiovascular disease. Include some relaxation in your daily routine. This may be yoga, tai chi, walking (preferably somewhere green), meditation or breathing exercises.

If there is one muscle worth looking after in the body it's your heart. Anything that raises the heart rate so you're breathing more deeply but still able to have a conversation is ideal. This may be brisk walking, cycling, swimming, jogging, skipping or dancing. Whatever it is enjoy it and do it regularly. Aim for between thirty and forty minutes five or six times a week. Exercise helps to lower blood pressure and cholesterol, dissipates stress hormones, burns calories, improves blood-sugar control and makes you feel good!

Get to the dentist. Studies have shown that people with gum disease may be at a greater risk of heart disease. Such harmful bacterial components in the blood can travel to other organs such as the heart, leading to atherosclerosis (narrowing of the arteries) and heart attacks. The supplement co-enzyme Q10 has been shown to help to prevent gum disease.

Dental problems

Dental problems such as tooth decay, periodontal disease and gingivitis can all increase as we age. A high percentage of post-menopausal women end up losing one or more teeth. This is often due to loss of alveolar bone – the bone that holds the teeth in the mouth. Loss of this bone may be due to reduced oestrogen and progesterone leading to some degree of osteoporosis. Periodontal disease is another cause. This usually starts with poor dental hygiene – a build-up of food and bacteria around the gums. This forms plaque and the plaque leads to bleeding, bad breath, inflammation and infection (gum disease or gingivitis). Infection can cause the bone supporting the teeth to break down. Abscesses as well as loose or lost teeth can result.

Dental diseases are increasingly being seen as early indicators of underlying health problems such as diabetes, osteoporosis and heart disease, so they're not to be taken lightly. Just remember they're highly preventable.

What you can do

Attend regular check-ups with your dentist and hygienist, floss daily and brush twice a day. A wise dentist once told me you only need to floss those teeth you'd like to keep!

Use natural, non-alcohol mouthwashes to help remove plaque and plaque-forming bacteria. Tea tree oil, grapefruit-seed extract, goldenseal and sage are all good antibacterial ingredients to look for. Alternate with a sea-salt water mouthwash (you can make your own).

There's a definite link between smoking and gum disease, as well as most other dental problems including oral cancer. Avoid nicotine gums, too.

Clove oil is a good medicine-cabinet basic for toothache and gum infections (buy it at the chemist). Apply it directly to the affected area on a sterile swab for pain relief.

Gillian's diet and supplement tips

Always consult a medical doctor before taking a course of supplements.

- Avoid fizzy drinks and acidic fruit juices and diets high in sugar and refined carbohydrates.

- Eat raw carrot and celery sticks. Chewing on these can help to strengthen the teeth and jaw.

- Fill up on vitamin C-rich fruit and vegetables. This vitamin is needed for healthy gums and has anti-inflammatory effects. Good sources include berries, green vegetables, currants, melons, peas, peppers, watercress and kiwi fruits.

- Eat a calcium- and magnesium-rich diet for healthy bones and teeth. Sources include almonds, figs, sesame seeds, green vegetables, quinoa, chickpeas, oats and haricot beans.

- Co-enzyme Q10 improves oxygenation of the tissues and aids healing. It is often low in those with gum disease. Suggested dose: 90mg a day.

- Take vitamin C plus bioflavonoids for good gum health and repair. (Make sure you get a buffered vitamin C as other types can be acidic and detrimental to tooth health.)

- Your teeth and bones are made of similar minerals so taking a bone-health formula will also benefit your smile. Look for one containing calcium, magnesium, vitamin D, boron, zinc and B vitamins.

Depression

The majority of women thoroughly enjoy life after the menopause and in later years, so please don't think a black cloud is about to descend on you – it's not! However, for some, depressed moods and general malaise may surface. This may not be diagnosed as clinical depression by your GP, but nevertheless it can significantly affect your quality of life.

A depressive state in later life may be due to the fact that our sex hormones have a profound effect on our neurotransmitters – the brain chemicals that affect our mood. These feel-good chemicals include serotonin and norepinephrine (noradrenaline), higher levels of which are associated with a positive mind state. It's thought that oestrogen increases the activity of serotonin and norepinephrine, boosting mood. With lower levels of oestrogen in the decades after the menopause, these chemicals are less active and the usual stresses of daily life may take their toll more than they would have previously. (And don't discount the emotional impact of empty-nest syndrome, if you have grown-up children who've recently left home – more on this on page 402.)

Depression can manifest itself in many ways: a lack of motivation; not finding pleasure in daily life; feeling low; a deep sadness; despondency; not being interested in doing anything; not feeling inspired by anything; mood swings; crying; lack of self-esteem; not being interested in food; weight loss or gain; self-blame for all kinds of things. Of course we all experience such states from time to time, especially after some sort of trauma. What counts as depression is when these symptoms don't appear to have a cause (such as bereavement, job loss or relationship break-up), or when they persist for more than a couple of weeks and interfere with your ability to lead a normal life.

Depressive moods are usually multi-factorial. Other than the hormonal changes described above, the following may also be exacerbating the situation:

- Liver stagnation
- Food sensitivities
- Vitamin deficiencies, especially the Bs
- Hereditary factors
- Adrenal fatigue
- Thyroid problems
- Medication
- Too much sugar in the diet
- Poor diet
- Alcohol excess
- Caffeine excess
- Low levels of tryptophan and serotonin (feel-good brain chemicals)
- Low blood-sugar levels
- Low hydrochloric acid

'Keep your brain firing by keeping it busy, stimulated and well nourished.'

What you can do

It's vital to talk to people if you're feeling low – even if it's the last thing you feel like doing. Many effective talk therapies, such as cognitive behavioural therapy (CBT) are now available from your GP.

In addition, both diet and lifestyle can play a major role in how you feel. So your main aim here is to correct nutritional deficiencies or imbalances and to support liver detoxification, the adrenal glands, the hormonal system and the nervous system.

Look at your diet and keep a food and mood diary for a week or so, to see if you can spot any connection between what you're eating (or not eating) and how you feel mentally and emotionally. Food has a huge effect on mood.

Gillian's diet tips

- Eat little and often: six small balanced meals a day to keep your blood-sugar level balanced and mood constant.

- Drink two litres of water a day. Vegetable juices are a good option, too.

- Eat tryptophan-rich foods. Tryptophan is an amino acid that converts to serotonin in the brain. It is found in brown rice, chicken, turkey, tofu, tempeh, fish and nuts.

- Carbohydrates may improve mood by aiding the transport of tryptophan into the brain, where it can be converted into serotonin. Stick to complex carbs – good sources include brown rice, quinoa, millet, buckwheat, oats, squash, sweet potatoes and polenta.

- Essential fatty acids (EFAs) are vital for good brain health, memory and mood. Increased levels of omega-3, a type of

EFA, have been found to reduce depression. They're found in oily fish, hemp seeds, pumpkin seeds, flaxseeds and their cold-pressed oils.

- Low thyroid function can be a catalyst for feeling low, so get this checked by your GP. And see my section on hypothyroidism, page 373.

- Certain fresh fruits help to stimulate energy flow through the liver, especially dark grapes, blackberries, strawberries, blueberries and raspberries. For optimum digestion, always eat fruit by itself, not with meals – in the morning is best.

- Foods high in chlorophyll such as spirulina, wild blue-green algae, wheat grass or barley grass, will supply your diet with essential fatty acids as well as vitamins and minerals needed for brain health and overall wellbeing.

- Sulphur is needed by the liver for detoxification, so include plenty of broccoli, Brussels sprouts, cabbage, cauliflower, onions and garlic in your diet.

- Green vegetables and leafy greens are good sources of magnesium, important for mood and energy. Grains containing magnesium include amaranth, millet and quinoa. Legumes include kidney beans, peas, soybeans and tofu.

- To look after your brain and mood, avoid added sugars, alcohol, caffeine and smoking – all of which may give the illusion of a temporary lift, but are ultimately mood killers. Diet and fizzy drinks contain chemical sweeteners and additives which may actually trigger depression.

- Nettle tea mid-afternoon is a great pick-me-up. My clients tell me they feel more energized and happier after just one cuppa. But feel free to drink a couple of cuppas. It's a nice afternoon lift and packed with nutrition.

Turkey meatballs with tomato sauce

Turkey contains tryptophan which converts to the mood-lifting serotonin in the brain. Combine with root vegetables, such as squash, sweet potoatoes, parsnips and carrots, which aids the transport of tryptophan into the brain.

SERVES 4

500g fresh turkey mince, preferably organic or free range
1 medium onion, peeled and finely chopped
1 plump garlic clove, peeled and crushed
1 small bunch (about 20g) fresh coriander, finely chopped
½ tsp organic 'wheat-free' vegetable bouillon (stock) powder

For the sauce

400g-can chopped tomatoes
1 garlic clove, peeled and chopped
1 medium onion, peeled and roughly chopped
1 celery stick, trimmed and thinly sliced
1 large carrot, peeled and thinly sliced
1 sweet potato, peeled and cubed
1 leek, trimmed and finely sliced
1 courgette, trimmed and cubed
1 bay leaf

1 Place all the sauce ingredients in a large saucepan. Fill the empty can from the tomatoes with cold water and pour over the vegetables. Bring to the boil, then reduce the heat and simmer gently for 25–30 minutes until the vegetables are tender and the sauce is thick, stirring regularly.

2 Meanwhile, preheat the oven to 200°C/Gas 6. Place the turkey in a large bowl and mix with the onion, garlic, coriander and bouillon powder.

3 Form the mince mixture into 20 small balls and place on a baking tray lined with foil. After 10 minutes, turn the meat balls. Return to the oven for a further 10 minutes until lightly browned and cooked through.

4 Allow the sauce to cool for 5 minutes. Discard the bay leaf and blend the sauce until smooth. Return to the pan and stir in the meatballs. Heat through gently until the sauce is hot. Serve with a crisp salad or the sweet potato rostis opposite.

Sweet potato rosti with cucumber salsa

SERVES 2-3 AS A STARTER
325g peeled and coarsely grated sweet potato
4 spring onions, peeled and finely chopped
1 garlic clove, peeled and crushed
2 tbsp chopped fresh coriander
1/2 tsp ground cumin powder
1/2 tsp organic vegetable bouillon (stock) powder
1 tsp poppy seeds
Virgin olive oil, for brushing
For the salsa
75g cucumber, diced
2 ripe vine tomatoes, chopped
1 tbsp chopped fresh mint
Handful of rocket leaves, lightly dressed in olive oil, to serve

1 Half fill a large saucepan with cold water and bring to the boil. Add the sweet potato and return to the boil. Immediately drain through a sieve and rinse under running water until cold. Line a large baking sheet with non-stick foil. Preheat the oven to 220°C/Gas 7.

2 Take handfuls of the sweet potato and squeeze any excess liquid into the sink – you need to remove as much of the liquid as possible. Transfer to a bowl and stir in the spring onions, garlic, coriander, cumin, bouillon powder and poppy seeds.

3 Take 2 heaped tablespoons of the mixture and press tightly between the palms of both hands to make into a patty shape. Place on the baking tray. Repeat with the rest of the mixture.

4 Brush the rosti lightly with oil and bake for 10 minutes. Carefully remove the tray from the oven and turn the cakes over using a spatula. Return to the oven for a further 10 minutes until lightly golden and crisp around the edges.

5 While the potato cakes are cooking, prepare the salsa. Place the cucumber, tomatoes and mint in a small bowl and mix well together. Serve the hot potato cakes topped with spoonfuls of salsa, accompanied by a few lightly dressed rocket leaves.

Supplement and herb tips

Always consult your medical doctor before taking a course of supplements and check with a herbalist for the correct dosage of herbs.

- Taking a daily vitamin B complex is a must. B-vitamin deficiency can lead to depression.

- Supplement with fish oils containing EPA and DHA.

- The amino acid L-theanine (found in small amounts in green tea) is excellent for fast relief of anxiety and inducing calm.

- The herb rhodiola is a great anxiety-reducer and antidepressant and results are usually noted within a few days. Take it at times of need rather than constantly – or try a two-weeks-on, two-weeks-off approach.

- The herbal plant milk thistle protects the liver from damage, enhances the flow of bile and fats to and from the liver, and improves the detoxification process. When the liver is doing its job properly you do feel better.

- St John's wort, often dubbed 'the sunshine herb' has been proven as an antidepressant. It is available as a supplement or as a tea. You must consult with your medical doctor before taking this as it can react badly with some medications.

- Ginkgo biloba fluid extract improves circulation to the brain, with positive effects on mood. Take the herb gota kola in conjunction with ginkgo for even better effect.

General lifestyle tips

Do aerobic exercise – something which gets your heart rate up so you feel a little breathless and sweaty – daily for at least twenty minutes. Build up gradually to more than that. My clients work up in stages to an hour a day. Exercise is great for improving blood-sugar control, brain chemistry, dissipating stress hormones and improving mood generally. Jogging, brisk walking, swimming, cycling, skipping and dancing can all make you feel better and improve overall health. In fact, exercise is now known to rival medication for its antidepressant effects, so much so that many GPs even prescribe it.

Get outside every day in natural daylight, whatever the season or weather (in fact make more of a point of doing this in winter, when it's tempting to hole up indoors all the time). Daylight is vital for normalizing body rhythms and moods. If you can exercise outdoors, all the better.

Learn to manage stress. If stress is a problem for you, then consider yoga, t'ai chi or meditation classes. Take time every day to do something that relaxes you, be it reading a novel, painting, having a bath or a massage.

Digestive problems

As we get older, problems with digestion may become more common. Many people produce less stomach acid and fewer digestive enzymes than they did previously. This can mean food is not fully broken down, so the bacteria in the gut are left to break down the partially undigested food molecules. One of the side effects of this is the production of gases with accompanying heartburn, bloating or flatulence. This, in turn, can contribute to constipation and irregular bowel movements. It can also lead to malabsorption, with symptoms of nutrient deficiencies such as skin, hair and nail problems, lack of energy, susceptibility to infections, slow healing, anaemia, weight loss or gain, depression, water retention, cravings and more.

Sometimes digestive disorders can result in seemingly unrelated symptoms such as headaches, fatigue and skin issues.

Chewing may be tricky if your teeth aren't as good as they once were. Saliva production may decrease with age and with lack of chewing. This is significant because saliva contains digestive enzymes that begin the breakdown of carbohydrates ready for more complete digestion in the small intestines. Gut bacterial imbalances are also more likely the older we get, due to years of poor diets, stress and use of medications.

Other factors that may contribute to digestive problems include, ulcerative colitis, coeliac disease, food allergies or intolerances, leaky gut, diverticulitis, Crohn's disease, irritable bowel syndrome, pathogens such as parasites and worms, stress, lack of physical activity, medications, laxatives, tea, coffee, alcohol, poor diet, surgery and cancer treatments.

What you can do

First of all, avoid placing undue strain on your digestive system by steering clear of foods that are hard to digest for many. These include red meats, fatty foods, fried foods, wheat and crisps.

If there are underlying problems behind your digestive issues, it's important to identify what these are and take the necessary steps to address them – otherwise you may put yourself at increased risk of many other conditions and complications. I'd advise seeing your GP.

And don't discount the importance of regular physical activity for good digestion – not while eating, of course! Walking, swimming, gardening – it all counts. Even some chair exercises or a simple stretching routine. Stretching increases blood circulation and oxygenation and is great for the digestive system, so have a good stretch twice a day.

Gillian's diet tips

- Smell your food and take time preparing it. The body gets ready to digest food when you first think about food, see food, smell food and prepare food.

- Chew each mouthful until it is liquid before you swallow. You will release the flavours and enjoy your food more as well as reaping the benefits physically. Chewing releases saliva in the mouth. Saliva contains enzymes that begin the digestion of starch. This reduces the workload lower down in the digestive tract. Chewing also increases the production and release of stomach acid and digestive enzymes needed to break food down fully.

- If you can't chew, blend your food. Having dental problems does not mean you have to live on ice cream and custard.

You can blend most foods into a soup or purée consistency. You can then mix this with the saliva in your mouth before swallowing.

- Avoid empty calories and foods that reduce absorption or remove nutrients from the body, such as alcohol, sugar, refined carbohydrates, caffeine, fizzy drinks, processed foods, junk food and anything to which you may be intolerant.

- Use herbs and mild spices to flavour your food. The aromas these release during chopping, cooking and eating stimulate your digestive juices.

- Use brightly coloured fruit and vegetables to tantalize your eyes and your taste buds. Think of the rainbow plate with yellow, orange, green, red and purple foods. Even if you don't get all colours into one meal, aim to eat a range of colours over the day.

- Drink vegetable juices daily. These provide highly bio-available nutrients that require little in the way of digestive enzymes for their absorption (organic vegetables are higher in nutrients and lower in toxins).

- Eat superfoods daily. Spirulina, blue-green algae and barley grass are all packed full of nutrients. Add them to juices or smoothies and mix well with your saliva before swallowing.

- Drink water and herbal teas between meals – too much liquid with meals dilutes digestive juices. Useful herbal teas include nettle (for its mineral content) and fennel, peppermint, chamomile and ginger for their digestion-enhancing qualities. Dandelion-root coffee is also great for stimulating the liver and getting digestive juices flowing.

Get tested for food intolerances if digestive problems persist. For some people dairy products are common culprits, as are wheat, eggs and orange juice. Some folks may even find they are sensitive to tomatoes and soya – so no need to overdo your intake. Go to www.gillianmckeith.info for information on food-intolerance testing.

Get plenty of fibre. Fibre is needed for proper movement of food and wastes through the gut. Without it, diarrhoea, constipation and poor gut function can result. Fibre also encourages the growth of the beneficial bacteria in the gut which are important for proper digestion and absorption. In particular, eat foods rich in oligosaccharides, such as chicory and artichokes.

Supplement and herb tips

Always consult your medical doctor before taking a course of supplements and check with a herbalist for the correct dosage of herbs.

Take digestive enzymes such as bromelain or protease with meals to give your body a helping hand. Start by taking one with each meal and increase if necessary.

Supplement with probiotics daily. These contain beneficial bacteria such as acidophilus which aid digestion, absorption and bolster immunity.

Herbal digestives such as Swedish bitters can be taken before meals to enhance digestion as well. Just put twenty drops in hot water and sip fifteen minutes before eating.

Facial hair

Light-coloured, soft, fine hair is not uncommon on a woman's face. However, as you age sometimes this hair becomes darker, thicker and more prolific. This is because, as levels of female hormones decline, the ratio of male to female hormones increases, meaning they may have more of an impact. Areas affected may include above the upper lip, the chin, jaw, cheeks and neck and, while there's nothing wrong with this, some women find it unsightly or feel it affects their self-confidence. As well as the ageing process, other imbalances may be at play, such as:

- Overproduction of male hormones (androgens)
- Increased sensitivity to circulating androgens
- Decreased oestrogens
- Polycystic ovarian syndrome (in women of reproductive age, see page 150)
- Other hormonal imbalances
- Obesity – fat tissue can produce androgens
- Genetic predisposition – this is more common in some ethnic groups than others
- Certain medications

What you can do

Take regular, moderate exercise. Exercise burns fat, improves the metabolism and gets the circulation flowing, all of which are good for your endocrine (hormone) system. While some women resort to hair-removal treatments such as waxing, laser treatments and electrolysis, you may be able to reduce or prevent the problem by balancing your hormones with diet, herbs and lifestyle measures.

Gillian's diet and supplement tips

Always consult your medical doctor before taking a course of supplements and check with a herbalist for the correct dosage of herbs.

- Try to stick within a healthy weight range.

- Keep blood-sugar balanced to keep insulin levels low. Insulin may increase susceptibility to problems with hormone androgens.

- Vitamin D improves the cells' response to insulin, meaning less insulin needs to be produced. Take a supplement and spend time outside every day. Vitamin D is formed by the action of daylight on the skin.

- Foods such as soya, flaxseeds, chickpeas, wheatgerm and fennel seeds have a mild oestrogenic effect which may help to balance excess androgens.

- If oestrogen deficiency is likely, herbs such as black cohosh and red clover can have a mild oestrogenic effect. Phyto-oestrogenic herbs contain weak oestrogens that may help to balance the body's own oestrogen levels. You can get these herbs in capsule and tincture form in a health-food store.

- Herbs such as maca and liquorice may also help to balance the endocrine system.

Female cancers

Breast cancer

One in nine women will develop breast cancer at some point, and it's the most common cancer in the UK, excluding non-melanoma skin cancer. But although it's on the increase, survival rates are rising slowly and steadily, probably due to increased breast awareness, earlier detection and improved treatment. Most cases occur in post-menopausal women. In addition to age, the following are possible risk factors:

- Starting your period at a young age (under twelve)
- A late menopause (after fifty-five)
- Having no children or having them late in life
- Not breast-feeding
- Taking the contraceptive pill or hormone replacement therapy (HRT)
- Being overweight (especially after the menopause)
- A strong family history of breast cancer
- Carrying a breast-cancer gene (although this is rare and accounts for fewer than 10 per cent of breast cancer cases)
- Eating a high-saturated-fat diet
- Regularly drinking more than one unit of alcohol per day
- Having dense breast tissue
- Having certain benign breast conditions such as atypical hyperplasia
- Radiation exposure
- Leading a sedentary life with little or no exercise

Performing regular self-checks for breast changes is essential. Always report any changes that are unusual:

- A lump in the breast or armpit
- Change in size or shape of the breast

- Nipple inversion or puckering
- A rash around the nipple
- Nipple bleeding or discharge
- Puckering of the breast skin
- Swelling of the arm
- Persistent breast pain
- Breast inflammation

Some research has found that women whose breasts suddenly become tender after starting HRT are more likely to develop breast cancer. If you experience this then consult your GP immediately.

Endometrial cancer

About eight in every 100,000 women are diagnosed with endometrial (also known as womb or uterine) cancer each year in the UK. It is the fourth most common female cancer. It is most common in post-menopausal women, particularly those in their sixties. Risk factors may include:

- Unopposed oestrogen – if oestrogen is not balanced with progesterone then womb cancer becomes more likely. This is why it is more common after the menopause when the body still produces some oestrogen but even less progesterone
- Genetics – a rare condition called hereditary non-polyposis colorectal cancer (HNPCC) can increase the risk
- Being overweight
- Insulin resistance or diabetes
- A high-fat diet
- Drinking three or more units of alcohol a day.
- Not having children
- Infertility due to ovarian failure or not ovulating each month

- Irregular bleeding during and after the menopause
- A late menopause
- Not having periods
- Starting your periods early
- Endometrial hyperplasia in which the lining of the womb becomes thickened
- Polycystic ovarian syndrome
- Taking tamoxifen or raloxifene as part of treatment for breast cancer

The following may be early symptoms of womb cancer and should always be reported to your GP. But be reassured that many of these symptoms are common and are more likely to be due to a less serious condition:

- Post-menopausal bleeding
- Bleeding between periods
- Unusual vaginal discharge
- Loss of appetite

Ovarian cancer

As you age, the amount of the hormones oestrogen and progesterone produced by the ovaries diminishes and the risk of cancer increases. Ovarian cancer is the fifth most common cancer in women, after breast, bowel, lung and womb cancers. Five out of every hundred cancers diagnosed in women are ovarian cancers. Over 85 per cent of ovarian cancers are in women over the age of fifty. As well as age, risk factors include:

- A family history of cancer
- Having had breast cancer or endometriosis
- Fertility treatment or HRT
- Starting periods early or having a late menopause (after fifty-five)
- Being overweight or tall
- Smoking
- Eating a diet high in saturated fat
- Using talcum powder

For a long time ovarian cancer was dubbed the 'silent killer', as it was thought there were no early symptoms. However, doctors now know many women experience symptoms in the early stages, when the cancer is most treatable. Obviously, many of the following symptoms may also indicate much more minor problems, such as pre-menstrual syndrome or irritable bowel syndrome. However, it's important to report any of them to your GP if they're unusual for you, come on suddenly and/or are persistent.

- Pain or swelling in the abdomen
- Feeling bloated and uncomfortable
- Feeling full after eating small amounts
- Irregular periods, if you still have them
- Lower back pain
- A frequent need to pass urine
- Changes in bowel habits such as constipation or diarrhoea
- Pain during sex
- Tiredness
- Loss of appetite
- Nausea or sickness
- Shortness of breath

Female cancers – what you can do

My action plan may help you to boost your immune system, cleanse your body and balance your hormones – important factors in both preventing and fighting female cancers. If you are being treated for cancer, a good diet and lifestyle really are essential and will help you to cope better physically and emotionally. Just make sure you check with your GP before taking any of the suggested supplements.

The incidence of many hormonal cancers varies dramatically in different parts of the world. For instance, breast cancer is six times more common in the UK and US than in Japan. However, when women move from low- to high-risk countries, over time they acquire the same risk as women in the country they have moved to. This strongly suggests that dietary, lifestyle and environmental factors affect your risk.

Gillian's diet tips

- You need to keep your body cleansed and hydrated, so drink at least eight glasses of pure, filtered or mineral water daily.

- Eat fresh fruit and vegetables (preferably raw) every day – seven to nine portions are ideal. A rainbow of colours will help to ensure you get a variety of phytonutrients – powerful plant antioxidants that help to protect the body against cancer. Freshly pressed fruit and vegetable juices are concentrated in cancer-fighting antioxidants and help the body to cleanse and revitalize.

- Make vegetables from the cruciferous family your friends – these include broccoli, cauliflower, Brussels sprouts, cabbage, kale, turnips, swede and watercress. They contain a substance called indole-3-carbinol (I3C), which stimulates the conversion of oestrone, the form of oestrogen that is higher during the menopause and promotes breast cancer, into an inactive form. Indole-3-carbonil, is metabolized into di-indolylmethane (DIM) in the body. This has been found to have anti-proliferative effects on breast tissue and to reduce the development of breast cancer tumours.

- Flavonoids and isoflavones from fruit, vegetables and pulses have been shown to have a protective effect against the development of ovarian cancer.

- Diets high in meat and fat have been associated with an increased risk of ovarian cancer.

- Sprouted seeds and legumes are beneficial, especially broccoli seeds as they contain sulforaphane glucosinolate, a precursor to sulforaphane, in amounts up to fifty times higher than those found in regular broccoli. Animal studies show sulforaphane blocks the formation of mammary tumours.

- You need fibre-rich foods. Researchers have found a high-fibre diet reduces the risk of many cancers. Good sources include brown rice and other whole grains, wholemeal bread, muesli, oats, and beans and pulses.

- Foods that contain phyto-oestrogens are useful – they're plant-based compounds that have mild oestrogenic effects. These can help to balance oestrogen levels if they are too low by raising them slightly and will help to reduce the effects if oestrogen levels are too high. Many studies have found this mechanism to be cancer-protective. You'll find them in soya products (such as soya milk, tofu, tempeh and miso), linseeds, celery, fennel, wheat, oats, chickpeas and lentils.

- Eat foods rich in calcium – women with higher intakes of calcium have a lower incidence of breast cancer. Calcium is found in quinoa, green vegetables, almonds, tahini, figs, dulse, hazelnuts, kombu and wakame.

- As ever, essential fats are exactly that – a must. Sources include shelled hemp seeds, flaxseeds, pumpkin seeds, sunflower seeds, walnuts, dark leafy green vegetables, avocados and unrefined vegetable oils such as flaxseed oil and extra-virgin olive oil. Never heat unrefined vegetable oils as they are unstable when exposed to high temperatures. Oily fish is a good source of omega-3 fats, but can contain environmental toxins, so don't exceed three portions a week.

- Processed foods should be avoided as these provide empty calories, little fibre and are packaged in potentially toxic packaging – none of which will help your body to cleanse and detoxify. Avoid refined sugar, and all foods that contain it, too. If you have a sweet tooth, satisfy it with fresh and dried fruit (unsulphured).

- A high salt intake is associated with an increased risk of some types of cancer. Use herbs and mild spices to flavour food instead – as a bonus, many of these have beneficial properties for the immune system.

- Cut out all dairy if you have been diagnosed with breast cancer. Cow's milk is very high in milk proteins which are often hard to digest. It also contains insulin-like growth factor (IGF-1) which stimulates the division and reproduction of cells to aid the growth of the calf. IGF-1 is produced in humans especially during puberty when it stimulates the growth of breast tissue. There is some evidence to suggest that women with higher levels of IGF-1 in their bloodstream may be at a greater risk of developing breast cancer.

- Alcohol is a known risk factor for many cancers, but particularly breast cancer – your risk increases for every glass you have a day. The liver helps to break down oestrogen, preventing excessive levels from accumulating in the body but alcohol compromises liver function.

- Caffeine has been associated with an increase in malignancies in pre- and post-menopausal women, so steer clear of tea, coffee and colas in favour of grain-based coffee substitutes and herbal teas such as nettle, fennel, chamomile, peppermint, ginger and rooibos.

- Watch your meat intake. Meat and dairy products may contain xeno-oestrogens, literally meaning foreign oestrogens (see page 104 in the Reproductive Years section) that may have a negative effect on the body's own oestrogen balance. This may be due to the use of hormones to stimulate growth and milk production in some farming methods. Vegetarian foods and meat and dairy products from organically reared animals may be less of a problem. Plus charred meat contains cancer-promoting compounds, as does non-organic meat which may contain residues of artificial hormones and growth hormones. Good vegetarian sources of protein include tofu, beans, lentils, quinoa, nuts, seeds, eggs and natural live yoghurt.

- Foods high in saturated fats such as fried foods, red meat and full-fat dairy products (butter, cream and cheese) are absolute no-nos. A high fat intake is associated with an increased risk of breast cancer as is cooking with vegetable and corn oils (cooking with olive oil and canola oil does not carry the same risks). A high-fat diet also increases the likelihood you'll be overweight or obese, which is linked to many cancers.

Foods that contain toxic trans fats, such as hard margarine, biscuits, cakes, crisps, pastries and processed foods are associated with an increased risk of chronic disease including cancer. Many manufacturers have banned them but always check labels for 'hydrogenated' or 'partially hydrogenated' fats or oils and avoid them!

Supplement and herb tips

There are studies to support the efficacy of the following, but always consult your medical doctor before embarking on a course of supplements and check with a herbalist for the correct herb dosage.

Beta-carotene, buffered vitamin C, vitamin E and selenium are all antioxidant nutrients which can help to protect the body against cancer-forming agents.

A daily vitamin-B complex may help to boost energy levels.

Vitamin D has been shown to help to deter the development of breast cancer.

Co-enzyme Q10, produced naturally in the body, helps cells to produce energy and acts as an antioxidant. It also stimulates the immune system.

Animal studies suggest that calcium D-glucarate lowers oestrogen levels in the body – an effect that may reduce some cancers.

Inositol hexaphosphate (IP6) has been reported to possibly have anti-cancer activity.

The herb milk thistle supports liver function and may slow the growth of breast-cancer cells.

- Siberian ginseng may help the body to recover from chemotherapy and radiation therapy more quickly.

- Echinacea, red clover and astragalus may help to support your immune system.

- Polyphenols (antioxidants) in green tea have been associated with a reduced risk of several types of cancers, including breast cancer.

General lifestyle tips

- Being overweight increases your risk of breast cancer, especially if you are post-menopausal. Oestrone and oestradiol, both cancer-promoting oestrogens, can be produced to excess by fat cells. Which is all the more reason to ...

- ... take more exercise! We know being active slashes your risk of most cancers. It keeps your weight, your circulation, heart and mind healthy and reduces stress. On average, women who regularly walk, swim, jog and cycle for between thirty-five and forty-five minutes five times a week are less likely to develop breast cancer than sedentary women.

- Get outside every day with some skin exposed, especially in winter. Vitamin D is manufactured in the body by the action of sunlight on the skin, and women with higher intakes of vitamin D have been found to have a reduced incidence of breast cancer.

- Reduce your exposure to xeno-oestrogens – chemicals that mimic oestrogen. Buy organic food, chemical-free toiletries and cleaning products, and avoid wrapping food in clingfilm.

- Don't smoke – smoking is associated with an increased risk of many cancers.

Hair loss or thinning

Thinning hair is not uncommon during or after the menopause and in the decades that follow. The hair on your head and pubic hair may both start to thin. Possible underlying causes may include:

- Reduced thyroid function which is common in women at this stage of life (see 'Hypothyroidism', page 373)
- Decreased female hormones and increased male hormones
- Some medications
- Nutrient deficiencies, particularly iron, B vitamins and protein
- Malabsorption – digestive function tends to weaken with age
- Extreme dieting
- Poor circulation
- Stress, illness or emotional upset
- Genetic predisposition

What you can do

Improve your circulation by taking regular exercise (increased blood flow to the hair follicles will boost their nutrient supply). Yoga is particularly good as it includes inverted postures in which the head is lower than the heart, allowing blood to flow to the hair follicles.

Gentle massage may also improve blood flow to the area. Combine one tablespoon of olive oil with fifteen drops of rosemary essential oil and massage this into the scalp. Rosemary has a warming effect that may improve circulation to the hair follicles. Or treat yourself to some Indian head massage sessions.

Use natural products on your hair, rotate your shampoo, use a soft brush rather than a comb and avoid heat treatments on the hair.

What and how you eat can also have an effect. Chew thoroughly and relax when you eat to ensure maximum digestion and absorption.

Gillian's diet tips

- Eat foods that contain phyto-oestrogens – naturally occurring plant oestrogens. These have a mild oestrogenic effect that may help to balance the post-menopausal hormones. Foods containing oestrogens include soya, yams, alfalfa sprouts, linseeds, beetroot, pomegranates and chickpeas.

- Include foods rich in B vitamins such as brown rice, quinoa, lentils, sunflower seeds, oats and green vegetables.

- Eat sprouted seeds such as sprouted quinoa – a source of food enzymes, vitamins, minerals and amino. You can grow this yourself using a sprouting kit.

- Sea vegetables are a rich source of vitamins and minerals needed for thyroid function and hair health. Try hijiki, kelp, dulse and nori.

- Eat two tablespoons of pumpkin seeds a day for their zinc content. Zinc is vital for many body processes, including hormonal balance and hair growth.

- Eat foods rich in iron such as lean meats, fish, eggs, figs, dulse, kelp, kombu, parsley, watercress, broccoli, cavolo nero, prunes, nettles and lentils.

- Make sure you get your essential fats, vital for healthy hair and hormonal balance. Include plenty of oily fish, flaxseeds, pumpkin seeds, hemp seeds, walnuts and avocados.

- Avoid foods and drinks that interfere with mineral absorption such as tea, coffee and wheat bran.

- Avoid sugar and refined carbohydrates as these increase insulin levels which can have a negative effect on the hair follicles.

- Use mild spices to improve circulation. Ginger, cinnamon, cayenne pepper and cumin may all have a warming effect.

Supplement and herb tips

Always consult your medical doctor before embarking on a course of supplements and check with a herbalist for the correct dosage of herbs.

- Take a B complex that contains biotin. B vitamins are vital for hair growth.

- Have your iron levels tested and, if you are diagnosed as being low in iron, then take an iron supplement.

- Take digestive enzymes with meals to ensure maximum nutrient absorption.

- The beneficial bacteria in the gut manufacture some B vitamins, so supplementing with probiotics may help.

- Oestrogenic herbs may also be helpful. These include red clover, black cohosh and dong quai.

- The herb maca may support the whole endocrine (hormonal) system and may stimulate the body to produce more of its own oestrogen.

- Add green superfoods such as spirulina, algaes and wheat grass to your smoothies.

Hypothyroidism

People with hypothyroidism have an underactive thyroid, meaning it doesn't produce sufficient quantities of thyroid hormones – thyroxine (T4) and tri-iodothyronine (T3). As these control our metabolic rate (the rate at which we burn up calories for energy) and body temperature, a deficiency can result in fatigue, weight gain, low appetite, feeling cold, a slow heart rate, weakness, constipation and depression. Other symptoms often associated with hypothyroidism include dry skin, yellowish skin, a goitre (swelling on the thyroid gland), hair loss, loss of the outer third of the eyebrows and brain fog.

The cause may be a lack of thyroid hormones or there can also be a problem with the conversion of thyroid hormones into their active form. Another contributory factor may be the presence of thyroid antibodies that suppress thyroid function. However, it's not known why any of these factors would occur. Lack of certain nutrients needed for thyroid hormone production is one contributory factor. Lack of exercise, food intolerances and disturbances in the rest of the endocrine system may also be involved.

Hypothyroidism is more common in older people, especially women. It affects 1.5 to 2 per cent of people over sixty. However, it can affect you at a younger age and when it does it often first presents during pregnancy, the perimenopause or post-menopause, when the balance between oestrogen and progesterone is in flux and may impact on thyroid function. These transitional states may also be times when the requirements for thyroid hormones are increased, meaning symptoms of hypothyroidism are more likely to become apparent.

Adrenal stress also affects thyroid function as high levels

of the stress hormone cortisol may affect the conversion of the thyroid hormones into their active form or the use of the hormones by the body cells.

Symptoms of insulin resistance, which also increases with age, also seem to coexist with hypothyroidism.

What you can do

Put a thermometer by your bed. When you wake in the morning, before you do anything else, put the thermometer under your arm and lie still with it there for 10 minutes. Record your temperature in this way for five consecutive days. If it is consistently below 36.5°C, then your thyroid may be somewhat underactive.

If yours is, or you suffer from any of the above symptoms, ask your GP to test your thyroid function. It is important that you get tested for T4, TSH and thyroid antibodies. They may order an ultrasound, especially if you have a goitre.

A permanently decreased metabolism as a result of hypothyroidism is conventionally treated by a lifelong prescription for thyroxine hormone tablets.

As well as supporting the thyroid it is important to use diet to support the adrenal glands, blood-sugar balance and the female hormones, as imbalances in these can all exacerbate thyroid problems.

And don't forget to exercise every day. Exercise stimulates the metabolism and gets the blood circulating to all areas. Yoga is particularly good as the inverted postures get the blood circulating to the thyroid gland in the neck.

Gillian's diet and supplement tips

Always consult your medical doctor before embarking on
a course of supplements.

- Drink eight glasses of pure water a day. Fluid levels are vital
  for the whole endocrine system, including the thyroid.

- Fresh fruit, vegetables, nuts, seeds, whole grains, pulses and
  fish contain the essential fats, B vitamins, zinc, vitamin C
  and magnesium necessary to support your adrenal glands.

- Eat sea vegetables at least three times a week. Sea vegetables
  contain iodine which is needed for the production of thyroid
  hormones. Kelp and nori are particularly useful. They can be
  bought as flakes and sprinkled onto soups and salads. Only
  small amounts are needed as too much can actually
  suppress thyroid function.

- Eat two to three Brazil nuts a day. They're one of the best
  sources of selenium, a mineral needed for thyroid function.

- Fibre helps to increase satiety, remove old hormones from
  the body and control blood sugar. Good sources include
  brown rice, quinoa, oats, rye, lentils, beans, fruit and
  vegetables.

- The gliadin in wheat can be toxic to the thyroid so is best
  avoided. Some people do better without the other gluten
  grains as well (rye, barley, kamut and spelt).

- Avoid raw cruciferous vegetables, soya and millet as they
  can all interfere with iodine uptake which negatively affects
  thyroid function. The cruciferous vegetables are fine if cooked,
  and fermented soya in moderation is OK (as in natto, miso,
  tempeh and tamari).

- Steer clear of sugar, refined carbohydrates, processed foods, alcohol, salt and caffeine.

- People with both diagnosed hypothyroidism and subclinical hypothyroidism are at an increased risk of developing insulin resistance and associated disorders such as cardiovascular disease. It is therefore wise to follow a blood-sugar-balancing diet that excludes sugar and refined carbohydrates.

- Try to avoid fluoride and chlorine as they're both chemically similar to iodine and can displace iodine in the thyroid. Fluoride is found in many toothpastes, tap water and tea. Chlorine is found in tap water and swimming pools. Filter your water and use fluoride-free toothpaste from the health-food shop.

- Take 500mg of L-tyrosine, twenty minutes before breakfast and lunch. This amino acid is needed for normal thyroid function.

- If you are on thyroid medication, do not take calcium supplements at the same time as you take your thyroid medication as calcium may interfere with the uptake of the thyroid hormones.

Note: Be aware that some foods and supplements can affect the absorption of thyroid medication: walnuts, soybean flour, cottonseed meal, iron supplements or a multivitamin containing iron, calcium supplements, antacids containing magnesium or aluminium – check with your GP.

Low libido

Although it is not inevitable, some women experience a reduction in their sex drive during and after the menopause and in later years. For many – and their partners, too, this is a natural occurrence in their relationship and not cause for concern. Others would prefer to enhance their libido, and there are many effective ways to do this. A reduction in desire may be due to reduced levels of sex hormones, particularly testosterone and oestrogen, which are the main hormones responsible for libido. Vaginal dryness can also make sex uncomfortable or painful, so less appealing. This is usually the result of lower oestrogen levels. Urinary incontinence or poor bladder control may also be a factor, as may compromised thyroid function. (See sections on urinary incontinence, page 398, and hypothyroidism, page 373.)

Emotional and psychological factors, such as depression or anxiety, may also influence sex drive. Post-menopausal women sometimes experience a dip in self-esteem. Not feeling sexy or attractive can reduce self-confidence and suppress sexual appetite.

The adrenal glands produce some sex hormones and once ovarian hormone output decreases, the sex hormones from the adrenal glands become more significant. This is one of the reasons why stress often dampens sexual desire.

Gillian's diet tips

Make sure you get your essential fats in daily. These are vital for hormonal balance and psychological health. Low-fat diets are the worst thing for your sex life. You'll find healthy good fats in oily fish, pumpkin seeds, shelled hemp seeds, sunflower seeds and flaxseeds.

- Foods associated with libido and love include pomegranates, figs, avocados, artichokes, asparagus, pumpkin seeds, apples, vanilla, almonds, figs and berries.

- If stress is an issue, support your adrenal glands. Nutrients needed for adrenal function include magnesium, B5, vitamin C and the essential fats. Magnesium is found in whole grains, nuts, seeds and green vegetables. Vitamin B5 is found in avocados, meat, fish, eggs, whole grains and pulses. Vitamin C is found in fruit and vegetables.

- Some foods contain phyto-oestrogens – plant chemicals that have a weak oestrogenic action in the body. If hormone levels are low, they can increase oestrogen. Good food sources include soya foods such as tofu and tempeh, linseeds, oats and chickpeas.

- Iodine is a mineral needed for ovarian and thyroid function. The thyroid can be implicated in low sex drive. Eating sea vegetables such as nori, kelp, dulse and kombu regularly may help to improve thyroid function. Speak to your GP about having your thyroid tested.

- Drink plenty of fluids such as water, herbal teas and vegetable juices. Staying well hydrated is important to prevent drying out of the skin and vaginal wall.

- Add ginger and a dash of cayenne pepper to your supper before sexual activity – they'll both enhance circulation to your genitals.

- Don't overindulge in nightshade vegetables: peppers, aubergines, tomatoes, white potatoes.

The kidneys have an important connection to the strength of your libido – your sexual essence is stored there. Burning the candles at both ends, poor food choices and going to bed late weaken kidney essence. Kidney-building foods include quinoa, aduki beans, kidney beans, black beans, salmon, trout, fennel, onions, mung beans, water chestnuts, walnuts, blackberries, mulberries, blueberries, parsley, celery, beetroots, fenugreek, garlic, ginger, dandelion and rose hips.

Libido-boosting dip

1 avocado
2 generous tsp cacao powder
1 banana
A big handful of dates (stones removed)

Blitz the lot with a squeeze of lemon to prevent oxidation.

All of these are purported to have aphrodisiac properties.

Supplement and herb tips

Always consult your medical doctor before embarking on a course of supplements and check with a herbalist for the correct dosage of herbs.

- Niacin enhances blood flow to the skin and mucous membranes which may intensify the female orgasm, making sex more enjoyable.

- The amino acid L-tyrosine converts to L-dopa in the body and this is needed for libido. Take L-tyrosine thirty minutes before food for maximum effects.

- Magnesium is a muscle and nerve relaxant and may improve blood flow to the genitals.

- Support the adrenal glands with Siberian ginseng, gotu kola, astragalus or rhodiola. These may all help to balance the adrenals and increase stamina and energy. Do not take these if you are on any medications.

- Black cohosh has hormone and mood-balancing properties and seems to enhance blood flow to the genitals. Studies show it may relieve vaginal thinning and dryness.

- Chasteberry or agnus castus was traditionally used by monks to help them remain celibate, but was perhaps an unwise choice. It's known for its ability to balance hormones and boost sex drive, certainly in women.

- Damiana has a stimulating effect on the genitals and may boost blood flow to the area, increasing sensitivity. It's useful for both women and men with low sex drive linked to anxiety.

- Red clover contains isoflavones which have a mild oestrogenic effect and so may relieve vaginal dryness.

- The aptly named horny goat weed contains testosterone-like substances that increase desire in women and men (as well as goats!).

- Liquorice contains isoflavones that mimic the effect of oestrogen and progesterone, increasing desire and energy.

- Schisandra is commonly used by Taoist women to boost their sexual energy and increase vaginal secretions. It has powerful hormone-balancing properties and helps the body in times of stress.

- Wild pink yam has been used for centuries to enhance sexual vigour. Its natural, hormone-like substances help to regulate imbalances and act as a muscle relaxant, making sex more pleasurable. It also alleviates vaginal dryness.

- Avena sativa has long been thought to free up testosterone in both men and women making it more available for use.

- Saw palmetto is also useful for some women if low testosterone is a problem.

General lifestyle tips

- Use vitamin E to lubricate the vagina. Pierce a vitamin E capsule and apply the oil around the whole area.

- Aloe vera gel can also be applied topically to the vaginal wall. It is soothing and healing.

- Take time to be intimate with your partner, even if it's not going to lead to sex. Spend quality time together, hold hands, have romantic nights out, hug and massage each other.

- If stress is an issue, learn relaxation techniques such as meditation, breathing exercises, yoga or t'ai chi.

- Aromatherapy can be wonderful to boost mood, raise self-esteem and create a relaxing, sensual atmosphere. Aphrodisiac oils include bergamot, neroli, sandalwood, patchouli, jasmine and ylang ylang. Use them for massage, baths or in a vaporizer.

- Exercise is vital for improving your mood, self-confidence, physical health, appearance and circulation to the sex organs. Get moving daily in whatever way you enjoy.

- To boost kidney energy, take a twenty-minute power nap between three and seven o'clock in the afternoon. Lie on top of a hot water bottle at night.

- If the problem is psychological rather than physical, relationship or psychosexual counselling may help.

Osteoarthritis

Osteoarthritis (OA) is sometimes called 'wear-and-tear arthritis', and is a condition in which the cartilage on the ends of your bones, between joints, wears down. It becomes rough, resulting in friction, pain and inflammation and stimulating the overgrowth of bone cells as the body tries to correct the imbalance. This can lead to bony spurs and further pain.

It's usually the wrists, hands, knees, spine and hips that are most affected, and symptoms can include pain, stiffness, swelling, immobility and even deformed joints. Many people report feeling better in warm, dry climates and worse if it's cold and damp.

OA tends to strike people in their fifties and more than half of all people over sixty-five have some degree of OA.

Many more women than men get OA, particularly after the menopause. This may be due to the protective effects that oestrogen and progesterone exert on the skeletal system.

What you can do

I've seen many clients respond well to a better diet, supplements and lifestyle advice – even debilitating symptoms can be relieved to some degree. Most important is to work out if any foods seem to trigger OA flare-ups, so keep a food and symptom diary for a month or so. In my experience, wheat, dairy, eggs and chocolate are common culprits. Eliminate any foods that seem suspect to you for at least two weeks and see if it makes a difference. Reintroduce the food slowly and monitor any reactions – you may like to see a nutritionist to help you with this. Also crucial is to increase your intake of anti-inflammatory foods.

Gillian's diet tips

Increase your intake of oily fish, such as salmon, mackerel, sardines, pilchards, herrings, trout and halibut. These contain the anti-inflammatory omega-3 essential fats, EPA and DHA. Eat plenty of nuts and seeds, too – especially walnuts, pumpkin seeds, flaxseeds (linseeds), hemp seeds and their cold-pressed oils.

Fruit and vegetables are high in anti-inflammatory nutrients and can help to alkalize the body (arthritis is often a sign of acidity). Eat two to three pieces of fruit a day between meals on an empty stomach, plus two to three portions of vegetables with lunch and dinner. Some should be eaten raw. If cooking, try steaming, baking, roasting or water stir-frying rather than boiling them to within a centimetre of their lives.

- Some people find that eating citrus fruits exacerbates the problem.

- Green vegetables contain vitamin K and folic acid, needed for healthy bone and cartilage formation.

- Fresh pineapple, especially the core, contains the enzyme bromelain that can help to reduce inflammation.

- Alfalfa sprouts are a good source of healthy-bone minerals. You can even grow your own if you like.

- Sulphur is needed for the repair of cartilage and bone and helps your body to absorb and use calcium. You'll find it in asparagus, eggs, garlic and onions.

- Whole grains, such as whole grain brown rice and rye contain histidine which can remove excess metals from the body. People with arthritis often have high levels of copper and iron.

- Fibre from whole grains, flaxseeds and pulses help to remove waste from the body.

- Kombucha tea contains many important nutrients and enzymes that can improve mobility and reduce pain.

- Go easy on members of the nightshade vegetable family: potatoes, peppers, chillies, aubergines, tomatoes and tobacco. They contain a compound called solanine which promotes inflammation in some people.

- Watch your fat intake: saturates (in meat, dairy products and most ready meals and processed foods) can have an inflammatory effect. Definitely avoid processed meats such as ham, bacon, salami, sausages, burgers and the like, as well as margarines and hydrogenated fats.

Tea, coffee, wine and spinach contain oxalic acid which can increase acidity and worsen inflammation.

Salt, sugar, refined carbohydrates and processed foods can all be detrimental to health and increase weight and inflammation.

Supplement and herb tips

Always consult your medical doctor before embarking on a course of supplements and check with a herbalist for the correct dosage of herbs.

Countless studies have shown daily supplements of glucosamine and chondroitin sulphate are useful in relieving the pain of OA. Try them for three months and if you are finding them helpful, continue. If they are not helping, stop.

Take a daily fish oil or borage supplement. EPA, DHA and GLA essential fatty acids are all powerful anti-inflammatories.

Magnesium, boron and vitamins K and D all help your body to use calcium and may prevent the build-up of bony spurs between joints. Vitamin D is formed in the body on exposure to sunlight, so spend plenty of time outdoors.

Vitamins C and E have anti-inflammatory and protective effects.

Zinc is often low in those with arthritis and a valuable nutrient for immune function and repair.

It's worth taking a daily probiotic and/or digestive enzyme to help your body to digest and absorb nutrients.

Cat's claw can reduce the pain of arthritis.

White willow, black cohosh and meadowsweet all contain anti-inflammatory, pain-relieving salicylic acid.

The herbs burdock root, celery seed, devil's claw, horsetail, nettle, wild yam root, comfrey root, ginger and parsley may all be useful for easing OA.

General lifestyle tips

It's a myth that people with OA should avoid weight-bearing exercise. In fact, while high-impact activity is best avoided, regular, moderate activity is essential to strengthen the muscles and ligaments that surround joints and keep you mobile. Walking and swimming are suitable for most people. Obviously don't persist with something that causes you discomfort.

Carrying extra weight puts strain on your joints and can cause further damage, so try to lose any excess.

Physiotherapy, chiropractic and osteopathy can be useful to relieve pain and increase mobility.

Creams containing glucosamine, chondroitin, ginger or capsicum, rubbed into affected joints, may ease aches and pains.

Elevate swollen joints and apply cold packs to bring down inflammation.

Osteoporosis

Osteoporosis means 'porous bones' and affects a staggering one in three post-menopausal women in the UK (and one in twelve men). Commonly known as brittle-bone disease, it occurs when the inner mesh of bone, which resembles a sort of honeycomb, develops larger and larger holes, making the bone fragile and prone to fracture. For many women, the first sign that they have the condition is when a fracture occurs – often after a relatively minor mishap. Another indication is curvature of the spine, sometimes referred to as 'dowager's hump'. Although the whole skeleton can be affected, the bones of the wrist, spine and hips are most vulnerable.

Bone is living tissue and its inner mesh, which consists primarily of protein, calcium and other minerals, is self-regenerating. Old bone is constantly being broken down by cells called osteoclasts and replaced with new bone by cells called osteoblasts which stimulate the growth of new bone. Bone density usually peaks at about the age of thirty-five, after which time it starts to decline as part of the normal ageing process. That's why it's so crucial to build strong bones in adolescence and during your twenties.

So what predisposes people to developing osteoporosis? Various risk factors are thought to contribute, including:

- Lack of vitamin D, calcium or magnesium earlier in life
- A generally poor diet or malabsorption
- Smoking
- Coeliac disease
- Prolonged use of antidepressants or antacids containing aluminium
- Genetic predisposition

- Inflammatory bowel conditions
- Lack of exercise, especially weight-bearing
- Being underweight or anorexic
- Amenorrhoea (the abnormal absence of periods for any length of time)
- Being female
- Being post-menopausal
- Being on steroid treatments for more than three months
- Hyperthyroidism
- Diabetes

A note about these final two factors. The decline in circulating oestrogen and progesterone as we age can lead to reduced bone density. The reason? Because these hormones have a protective effect on bone health. Oestrogen inhibits osteoclasts while progesterone stimulates osteoblasts. Oestrogen also improves calcium absorption (a bone-health essential) and reduces calcium excretion in urine. So your requirements for calcium after the menopause are far greater.

What you can do

It's never to late to start looking after your bones, whether you've been diagnosed with osteoporosis, think you may be at risk or just want to prevent it at any age. After the age of about thirty-five, the goal is to slow the rate at which bone mass is lost.

Your main aims are to provide essential nutrients needed for healthy bone formation, to maximize absorption and minimize losses through the urine and other mechanisms. You also want to optimize hormone levels and to live a bone-healthy lifestyle.

Gillian's diet tips

> Plant-based diets have been found to reduce the risk of developing osteoporosis, perhaps thanks to their alkalizing effect on the body which may reduce the breakdown of bone. So that's yet another reason to eat plenty of fruit and veg – which are also rich in potassium, vitamin C and boron, needed for healthy bones.

> Green vegetables contain magnesium, as well as calcium and vitamins C and K, all of which are vital for healthy bones. Without magnesium, calcium cannot be absorbed into bone.

> Snack on nuts and seeds – excellent sources of calcium – and other bone nutrients, particularly almonds, hazelnuts, sesame seeds and raw shelled hemp seeds.

> Seaweeds, such as wakame, kombu, nori and agar, are also rich in calcium. Try mixing them into soups, broths and stews. Wakame is known as the 'woman's seaweed' thanks to its calcium content – try it in sandwiches instead of lettuce. Seaweeds also nourish the thyroid gland, which plays a role in controlling bone turnover.

> Beans and quinoa are not only rich in calcium but excellent protein sources, too.

> Essential fats are vital for healthy bones. Good sources include oily fish, pumpkin seeds, raw shelled hemp seeds and sunflower seeds.

> Phyto-oestrogen-rich foods may help to reduce the rate of bone loss, so include soya such as tofu, chickpeas, lentils and linseeds.

> Figs contain magnesium, calcium and phosphorus so they make a good bone snack.

- Soak rolled oats overnight in water and eat raw in the morning (try them mixed with some fruit, nuts and soya yoghurt to make a muesli). They contain silica, important for bones.

- Vitamin K helps to regulate bone metabolism. It has two forms in nature: vitamin K1 and vitamin K2. Vitamin K1 is found in broccoli, cavolo nero, savoy cabbage, Brussels sprouts, asparagus, avocados, spinach and nettles. Vitamin K2 is made in the intestines by the beneficial bacteria and is also found in fermented foods such as miso, natto and yoghurt as well as meat and eggs.

- Limit your meat intake, as its digestion leaves acid residues in the body that need to be neutralized with alkalizing minerals such as calcium, magnesium and potassium – diverting them away from your bones.

- Salt and sugar both increase the excretion of minerals and decrease the absorption of calcium in the body. Never add them to food and look out for 'hidden' sources in breakfast cereals, processed foods and confectionery.

- Coffee and alcohol may increase calcium excretion in the urine. Alcohol interferes with protein and calcium metabolism and affects bone-building cells. And fizzy drinks are well-known to leach vital minerals from bones, thanks to the phosphoric acid they contain. Stick to water and herbal teas.

Supplement and herb tips

Always consult your medical doctor before embarking on a course of supplements and check with a herbalist for the correct dosage.

- Take magnesium supplements or magnesium/calcium supplements where the magnesium ratio to calcium is higher. Calcium citrate/malate is the best form. You need around 1,500mg calcium daily from the menopause onwards.

- You'll also need vitamins D, B3, B6, B12, folic acid, C and K, manganese, boron and silica. Look for a bone-health supplement that contains all or most of these.

- If the bone formula does not include vitamin D then you ought to take that supplement separately. Suggested dosage: 400–800IU daily.

- Take digestive enzymes with meals to make sure that you are absorbing nutrients and breaking down food efficiently.

- Also take plant-based hydrochloric-acid supplements before meals. Most post-menopausal women are often low in the stomach acid needed to break down protein and release minerals from food.

- The herb horsetail is a source of silica for calcium metabolism.

- Drink ginseng tea and nettle tea, too.

General lifestyle tips

- Do not smoke. Smoking prevents mineral absorption needed for healthy bones.

- If you're on antidepressants or antacids, you must pay even more attention to your bones. Studies have found older people who take antidepressants and other drugs are more likely to break a hip than those who don't. All the more reason to take exercise and a good bone-building formula.

- Get outside for at least thirty minutes every day. Vitamin D is formed by the action of daylight on the skin and is vital for the retention of calcium as it stimulates calcium absorption in the gut.

- Exercise is one of the most effective ways of building bones, but it needs to be weight-bearing exercise, not just cardio. This means anything in which you're either lifting some sort of weight (such as at the gym or in a class), or you're supporting your body weight as you exercise, so you're asking your muscles to work harder than they normally would. Good weight-bearing forms of exercise include using resistance training machines or free weights in the gym, aerobics, walking, jogging, skipping, Pilates and yoga. (Swimming and cycling aren't weight-bearing.)

- If an exercise becomes easy, that's great – you're getting fitter and stronger. But now it's time to up the intensity, to work harder, longer or more often. Progression is key.

- Recent research has shown that regular sessions of weight-bearing exercise, coupled with 1,500mg of calcium and 400–800IU of vitamin D daily, can stop bone loss for some post-menopausal women.

- If you already have osteoporosis, be very careful with the weight-bearing exercise you do – seek the advice of your GP and a physiotherapist.

- Natural progesterone cream from wild yam may help to slow down bone loss.

Rheumatoid arthritis

Rheumatoid arthritis (RA) is a chronic, inflammatory autoimmune disease – where the body attacks its own tissues and cells. It causes joints to become inflamed, swollen and painful – so much so that they may eventually become deformed. The condition seems to start gradually in the small joints of the hands, wrists, feet, elbows, hips, knees or shoulders. Skin can also turn ruddy or purple over the affected areas. The condition may also cause general malaise, tiredness and loss of appetite.

There are many indicators to suggest that RA is, at least in part, influenced by female hormones – three-quarters of all sufferers are female (when men are affected, it tends to be more severe). Although it can develop at any time, it's most likely to develop once your natural hormone levels start to decline.

Women who have never had a child may be more likely to develop RA than those who have. Sufferers who get pregnant often find the disease improves during the pregnancy, when oestrogen and progesterone levels are high, but gets worse after the birth when hormone levels drop. Women with RA may find it more difficult to get pregnant and may be more at risk of osteoporosis.

Other, non-hormonal causes of RA are thought to include:

- Hereditary predisposition
- Food allergies
- Abnormal gut and bowel permeability
- EFA and GLA deficiency
- Smoking
- Chronic stress
- Vitamin D deficiency

What you can do

Diet can make a huge difference with RA – the more
vegetarian-based, the better. In fact I've seen clients respond
amazingly to a vegan diet (no dairy, meat or fish) or one that's
almost vegan, but includes some fish. Keep a food diary for a
month and see just how much meat, poultry and dairy you're
consuming – as well as wheat, potatoes, peppers, paprika,
tomatoes, fizzy drinks and caffeine. If it's a significant
amount, I'm sure you'd benefit from eliminating them.

Gillian's diet tips

- Eat plenty of fruit and vegetables for their antioxidant
  content. Particularly useful are yellow veg, such as squash,
  carrot and yams, and cruciferous varieties such as kale,
  cabbage, collards and Brussels sprouts (rich in a compound
  called molybdenum which helps the liver to detox).

- Enjoy berries for their flavonoids which may help to reduce
  swellings. Papaya is a wonderful anti-inflammatory fruit.

- Chomp on celery stalks and drink celery juice (if you don't
  like the taste, mix it with carrot, kale or cabbage juice).

- It's thought ginger may block the prostaglandins that cause
  inflammation. Use ginger in your cooking and in your veggie
  juices, too.

- The spice turmeric contains the flavonoid curcumin which
  has anti-inflammatory properties, and it's great in stews.

- Cayenne contains capsaicin which is thought to block pain.

- Get more oils into your body – so eat oily fish like salmon,
  herring, mackerel and sardines, use olive oil and gold-of-
  pleasure seed oil liberally on your salads.

- Sprinkle flaxseeds on your porridge – they contain anti-inflammatory fats as well as having phyto-oestrogenic effects which may be beneficial if low oestrogen levels are exacerbating the problem.

- Eat raw shelled hemp seeds for snacks and mash them into avocados.

- I'd strongly recommend avoiding all junk foods, fizzy drinks, pies, pastries, cakes and biscuits. Make your own treats and you'll know what's in them.

- In my experience, people with RA benefit from avoiding gluten – so steer clear of wheat, rye, oats, bulgur wheat, couscous and spelt. Gluten-free grains to choose instead include amaranth, buckwheat, millet, quinoa and rice. If you have to use a grain with gluten, sprout it.

- Try eliminating oranges and their juice as well as the nightshade family of vegetables. This includes potatoes, tomatoes, paprika, aubergines, bell peppers and, of course, tobacco. Some people are sensitive to a substance these contain called solanine, which interferes with the enzymes in the muscles, causing pain and discomfort. Solanine is also a calcium inhibitor and arthritis sufferers may be deficient in calcium.

- Try food combining to maximize digestion. That means fruit by itself, never for dessert, and not mixing dense proteins such as chicken or fish with dense carbohydrates such as potatoes or rice at the same meal.

- It's well worth seeing a nutritionist to be tested for food allergies and parasites.

Supplement and herb tips

Always consult your medical doctor before embarking on a course of supplements and check with a herbalist for the correct dosage of herbs.

- Ask your GP about the possibility of having vitamin B12 injections.

- Take a vitamin B complex (with extra B5) three times daily. The B vitamins are important because a deficiency may be a possible risk factor for RA.

- Take vitamin E daily in capsule form.

- If your arthritis is worse in winter, you could have a vitamin D deficiency (most people do!). It's a good idea for everyone to supplement with D in the winter, especially if you have little exposure to sun at other times of the year.

- Two tablespoons of flax oil daily would be of enormous benefit (simply swallow it, or you can add it to salads or smoothies). Or, if you're not following a vegan diet, take a fish-oil supplement.

- Take a beneficial bacteria (probiotic) daily for better gut function and nutrient absorption.

- See a nutritionist to obtain advice on how to improve digestion and absorption.

- Supplements of quercetin and celery-seed extract both have anti-inflammatory properties. Take them between meals.

- The herb yucca, in extract or capsule form, can be very helpful in combination with devil's claw.

> Take borage oil capsules, three times daily.

> Astragalus extract is good source of the B vitamins.

> The Ayurvedic herb boswellia may also be useful.

General lifestyle tips

> Many people report benefits from wearing magnetic bracelets.

> Adding apple cider vinegar to your bath water is an age-old remedy for soothing arthritic aches – a couple of tablespoons should suffice.

> Try to have regular body massage and try self-massage on your joints – use creams or oils containing ginger or capsaicin.

> Indian head massage may improve circulation in the brain, influencing the pituitary gland and hormone release.

Urinary incontinence

People with urinary incontinence are unable to fully control the emptying of the bladder. Anxiety, heavy lifting, exercise, laughing, coughing and sneezing may all trigger the release of a few drops or more of urine from the bladder.

The condition can be particularly common in menopausal and post-menopausal women whose oestrogen levels are on the decline. This leads to a loss of elasticity in the tissues, reduced blood flow to the pelvic area and weakened pelvic-floor muscles. The muscles may not have the strength to control the closing of the exit from the bladder, leading to leakage of urine.

There are also several types of incontinence (and it's possible to have a combination of these types):

- Stress incontinence is caused by extra pressure being put on the bladder by sneezing, coughing, laughing, heavy lifting or exercise.

- Urge incontinence is the most common type in post-menopausal women. It leads to a sense of urgency when you need to urinate, meaning you have to rush to the toilet to avoid leakage.

- Overflow incontinence is a result of the bladder not being able to empty completely, leading to a frequent need to go to the toilet and often leakage.

As well as lack of oestrogen, the following may cause or predispose you to the condition:

- Childbirth
- Weak pelvic floor muscles
- Gynaecological problems

- Chronic constipation
- Obesity
- Strokes
- Smoking
- Stress
- Spinal injuries

What you can do

It's important to find the underlying cause of the problem, so do report it to your GP as investigations may be necessary. They may prescribe pessaries designed to hold the vaginal tissues up and away from your bladder, thus decreasing the pressure on the bladder. And they'll almost certainly tell you to practise pelvic-floor exercises daily. These involve isolating and contracting the muscles that control the flow of urine (imagine you're trying to stop mid-pee). Special cones and balls can also be used to retrain the pelvic-floor muscles in the same way. There's even a medical treatment that involves electrical stimulation of the muscles to train them to contract and strengthen. Occasionally, surgical treatment is necessary. However, there's plenty you can try before it gets to that stage.

If you're overweight, try to lose it as any excess weight on your pelvic floor will make recovery harder. And if you smoke, stop! Incontinence is one of the many problems associated with smoking.

Dilute cypress essential oil in a carrier of sweet almond oil and use it to massage into your lower abdominal area daily. You can also try to tone the area by alternating between hot and cold bursts with the shower head, and relaxing with a hot-water bottle or compress on your kidney area.

Gillian's diet tips

- Many people with urinary incontinence limit their fluid intake in order to reduce the problem. However, this leads to concentrated urine that may exacerbate the problem. Stick to water and herbal teas and increase your fluid intake gradually to eight glasses or mugs a day.

- Eat green foods that are high in calcium and magnesium needed for proper muscle and nerve contraction and relaxation. Other sources include almonds, hazelnuts, Brazil nuts, sesame seeds, sea vegetables, parsley, quinoa and oats.

- Drink barley water daily. Simmer half a cup of pot barley in five cups of water for twenty-five minutes. Add grated ginger and lemon juice for extra flavour. Strain and drink.

- Avoid salt, alcohol, caffeine, fizzy drinks, chocolate and spices. These may irritate a sensitive bladder.

- Acidic food and drinks such as tomatoes, orange juice and cranberry juice may irritate the bladder. (Interestingly, cranberry juice is beneficial for infections in the urinary tract, but may exacerbate incontinence.)

- Eat foods rich in oxalic acid – spinach, chard, rhubarb, eggs, asparagus, beet greens, sorrel – in moderation only.

Supplement and herb tips

Always consult your medical doctor before embarking on a course of supplements and check with a herbalist for the correct dosage of herbs.

- Higher intakes of vitamins B, D, calcium, protein and potassium have all been associated with decreased risk of incontinence.

Dear Gillian,

My thyroid was sluggish, and I was lacking specific vitamins. Just implementing the tools that you taught, on the holistic approach to proper nutrition, and of course exercise, I, my children and my husband are now eating more healthily, and the pounds are falling off! Thank you!

   Danielle

Dear Gillian,

By following the concepts and switching to the foods you recommended we've both lost weight, but more importantly, have become incredibly healthier! My wife's hair is shiny, her nails are strong, and her skin is becoming smoother. I no longer need the blood-pressure and cholesterol medications I was taking, and we're both healthier than we were thirty years ago.

   John and Chris

Dear Gillian,

In five months I have lost four dress sizes, have an average blood pressure of 110/68, have stopped taking meds for cholesterol, have had not one episode of diverticulitis and my bowels are amazing!!

   Everything that goes in comes out in a timely, pain-free manner. In other words, I am the master of my own body, health and wellbeing after sixty years of misery.

   Most sincerely,
   Karen

'Paying attention to your health now will pay huge dividends. Yes, you may have to work harder at exercise if you want to maintain that toned tush! Your diet may need significant adjustments if you want to avoid abdominal weight gain. But it can be done. Be extra aware, not extra worried. Think of those people you know, be they friends, family or celebrities, who seem to defy their age. I'll bet that's not due to the surgeon's knife or a Botox habit, just good, clean living!'

Q: Dear Gillian,

The youngest of my three children has just left to go to university, so now it's just me and my husband at home. I thought I'd relish the free time this would give me – less washing, fewer meals to cook, a tidier house. I was expecting a second youth for my husband and me. Instead, I've been feeling very low, as if life doesn't have a point any more. Should I be feeling like this?

Dorothy, 57

A: Dear Dorothy,

It sounds to me very much as if you're experiencing empty nest syndrome. It is not uncommon for women (and sometimes men) to feel a sense of emptiness when their offspring leave home. It is perfectly normal to feel sad or weepy and it is best to allow yourself to experience these emotions. You are likely to have friends or relations who have been through similar experiences so share your feelings with them. I am sure they will be very understanding.

It's fine to tell your sons or daughters that you are missing them but it is also wise to let them enjoy their freedom and this new phase of their lives without guilt-tripping them about leaving you. Let them know that you are there for them whenever they need you but avoid coming across as needy. Arrange the best times and ways of communicating with them regularly. Phone calls, texts, emails and internet phone calls make staying in touch really easy. Let them know they are welcome to come home for weekends or special occasions whenever they like. You can visit them, too.

If your emotions are overwhelming and continue for months then consult your GP about counselling or support groups in your area. If there are problems with your relationship with your partner or if you have underlying health problems these could well be exacerbating your feelings so seek out relevant help.

Make sure that you eat properly and take care of yourself. Just because you are cooking for two or maybe even one, you must still make sure that healthy eating and exercise are a priority for you. Your mood and sense of wellbeing depend on it.

This is a natural time for you to re-evaluate your life and your place in the world. You are now free to pursue new interests. Think about what you have always wanted to do and do it! Make a life plan for yourself. Sign up for courses, go travelling, decorate the house, learn to paint or play an instrument. You can even start a new career or sign up for voluntary work. All of these can help you to feel fulfilled and satisfied with your life again. Your new interests will also make you a more interesting person so your grown-up children will be more inclined to want to spend time with you and to introduce their friends to you, too. In a way it's a whole new beginning and an exciting journey.

Conclusion

My goal when writing this book was for everyone who reads it to come to realize the 'specialness' of being a woman. Hopefully, I've managed to banish any negative beliefs you may have held about 'a woman's lot' or the inherent suffering and hormonal hell some would say is our gender's destiny. It. Is. Not!

Whether or not you've yet had a chance to put any of my advice into practice, I hope I have demonstrated that while we women may face certain specific health challenges, we have every chance of overcoming them. Health, vitality and energy in abundance are yours for the taking, so long as you nurture and prioritize yourself.

I can tell you unequivocally that if you refer to this book regularly, throughout your life, and implement my advice, then you are primed to:

- Minimize or eliminate ailments

- Give yourself the best chance of preventing illness in the first place

- Influence vitality, rejuvenation and a healthy and fulfilled future

After almost two decades studying, researching and teaching in the field of food and holistic nutrition, and working with clients in private practice, I know what works and what gets real results. And something that I truly hope has sparked your interest as you've read this book is my key belief that good health, a fit body and a fulfilled life are not achieved by food alone.

Of course, food is an essential foundation, but it is only one physical component of my approach. The whole picture comprises:

- The right foods

- Regular moderate exercise

- Energy synchronization

As I discussed in my introduction to this book – and as I have expanded upon when writing about each life stage – ultimate health means having your physical and metaphysical energies working in harmony. Food provides you with living, physical energy while your thoughts, emotions and spirit comprise your metaphysical energy. When both forms are primed and in balance, then you will feel well and have the best chance at preventing illness and eliminating health complaints.

Even if you are sceptical at this stage, or you're not sure you fully understand how to work with your energies, know this: Energy synchronization starts with the physical aspect of food. Good, nutritious, life-giving foods are of a high vibrational energy. Unhealthy junk foods are of a low vibrational energy. By eating the former – the foods I recommend throughout this book – you ensure that your cells, organs and body as a whole are of the highest vibrational energy possible.

When you're ready to move to the next level – and perhaps you already are – you can also follow the energy synchronization advice and exercises I give for different life stages. This brings in the metaphysical side. The combined approach is your route to ultimate health on all levels.

So, you see, while nutrition is the foundation of my approach, I want to give you so much more. I want to uncover to you the fullest picture in achieving not only good physical health, but balanced emotional, mental and spiritual health, too. So please continue to use this book as your women's health bible, your lifetime reference guide. But I would urge you also to open yourself to the ideas and practices of energy work that I describe. For they will set you firmly on the path to true health and happiness.

Lots of love and light,

Gillian

Index

Recipes index

Acknowledgements

Big thank you to Howard for his inspiration and vision.
Immense gratitude to Josie. Gigantic thanks to Hannah.
Gratitude to Laura and everyone at Penguin. Together,
we are helping to empower women everywhere to take
responsibility for their own health. Let's do one for the men!
And that reminds me, a big hug for you, Luigi. Warmest
wishes to all my clients over the years, and to my website
club members too. Finally, much appreciation to the many
millions of viewers who watch and support my television
shows around the world.

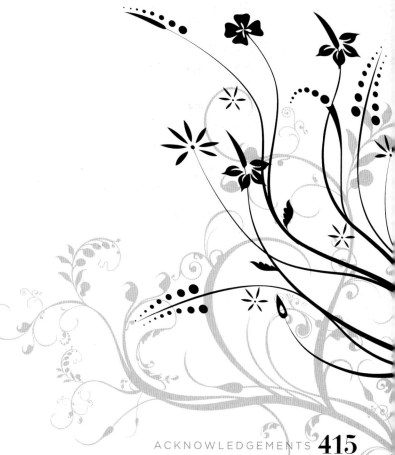

www.gillianmckeith.com

Get Gillian's ongoing support when you join
the club www.gillianmckeith.com

The Gillian McKeith Club includes:

- Personal Health Profile
- Meal Plans
- Weekly Top Tips
- Recipes
- Gillian's Boot Camp
- Club News
- Club Forum
- Research Centre
- Nutrition Clinic
- Newsletter
- Club Resources, Video Library and Archives
  And more!